I0705014

BIG UP MANHOOD:
Rites-of-Passage to Reclaim Masculinity and Restore Bio-Integrity

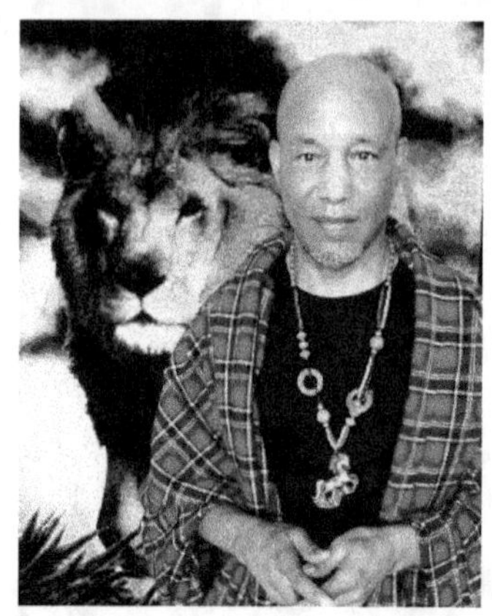

This book is authored by Keidi Awadu. and published by the Conscious Rasta Press for Black Star Media Global, Las Vegas, Nevada U.S.A. Copyright 2023

Keywords: aging, bio-integrity, cardiovascular disease (CVD), culture, education, erectile dysfunction, exercise, fatherhood, gender, hormones, longevity, Low-T, masculinity, nutrition, prostate health, sperm health, testosterone, vegan & vegetarian

"We could not be Africans and slaves at the same time; we could not hold on to our African identity, our African selves, knowledge of our African culture, and be enslaved...the subordinates of another people.

It is only when that knowledge is removed, erased, degraded, stolen, taken and distorted that we lose our identity. It is then that our identity is placed upon us by another people and by external forces.

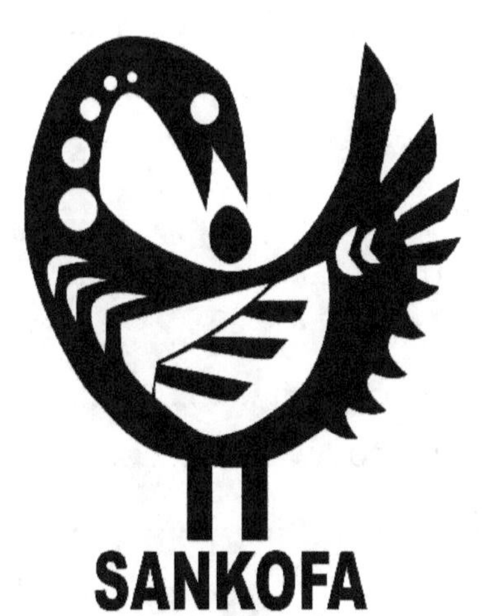

"Therefore a lack of self-knowledge is a lack of self-awareness is also an insensitivity to the self. But an insensitivity in the self is also an insensitivity to reality and to the outside. Without the sensitivity of the outside world and the self, we are left to blindly stumble from one point to another." – Dr. Amos Wilson[1]

---

[1] Cited in To Be Afrikan: Essays by Afrikan in the Process of Sankofa (Returning to our Source of Power, Volume 1, Edited by Burnett Kwadwo Gallman, Marimba Ani, Larry Obadele Williams, Maat Inc., 2003

Table of Contents

Introduction

Our backs were pressed against the wall. Our dilemma spiraled downward until it became an existential matter. That is when the Lions returned and engaged in the battle. We had no choice but to win! We recaptured our Pride from the hyenas that had for too long assaulted our families." – Keidi Awadu

The "Nature" of the Problem

"The Nature of a Man" is a phrase we have encountered numerous times within our communications and across community engagements. When writing or speaking on this theme, I am considering this analysis's biological, mental, and spiritual nature. We have a long legacy of musings on the concepts of manhood, gathered from our family experiences and the public commons we have encountered and inherited throughout our lives.

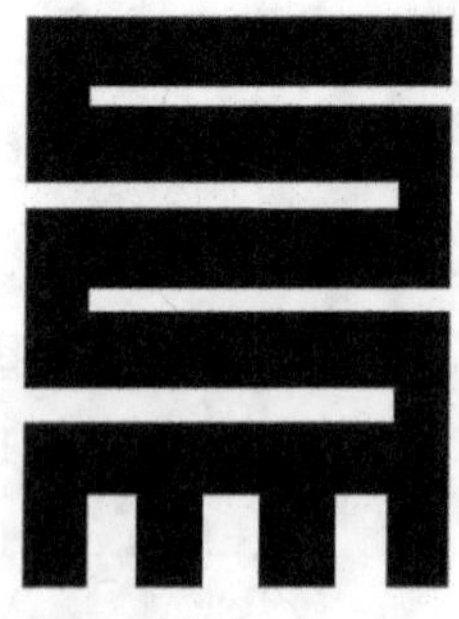

Nkyinkyim: the tortuous nature of life's journey

The community's outstanding men best define the Nature of Man. In addition, elders have a special place of authority in the evolution of Africans and other civilized groups throughout history. In such societies, older women are similarly given a special position of respect. They thus are expected to guide the decisions of the collective toward optimal outcomes of sovereignty and sustainability.

In civilized societies, these elders have invested their lives in learning, craftsmanship, providing valued services that benefit the group, growing food, building housing, creating mechanisms of security, cultivating land, and teaching subsequent generations to inherit, expand, and secure the grand enterprise. These patterns have existed since the dawn of civilizations, great and small. They must continue perpetually, or else the group is in peril of degradation, decay, and demise.

Wise words help us realize the profoundness of the question of the *nature of a man*.

- A man is the adult stage of a biological male, which is determined by three genetic features: his reproductive organs, glandular system, and brain structure.

- Man is a highly evolved mammalian of the primate subspecies.

- Man is reflective of the environment that has shaped his biology and personality.

- A man is impacted throughout life by both psychological and sociological inputs, which can often distort his masculine identity.

- Man exists as an integral component of and contributor to the society into which he has been groomed.

- From our African cultural perspective, Man is *essentially good*, as demonstrated in his affairs, actions, and morality.

- Man is, by Nature, a defender of those elements which create sovereignty and sustainability.

- In his mentally healthy state, Man is driven by logic and reasoning, in preference to emotionalism and being "feelings driven."

- Man is an innovator, creator, inventor, and protector.

- Man is inherently committed to perpetuating his kind for future generations; thus, he would self-sacrifice to preserve family and the future of the collective.

- Man is comfortable in a masculine alignment and has no interest in projecting himself in the world as feminine or *gender ambiguous.*

- Man has a strong drive to align with others like himself to protect and project mutual interests.

Throughout the course of this book, as an extension of our rites-of-passage, we will often return to defining the nature of Man.

Let's Distinguish Between a Male and a Man

In my honest opinion, society nowadays is getting a little more than a bit crazy – It's done gone BUCK WILD! People are making all kinds of claims about all manners of things. Conspiracy mongers are running amok. People are repeating incredibly wild claims such as:

- Shape-shifting lizard people from another galaxy are running societies;

- People are claiming to be magical shamans, wizards, warlocks, and witches;

- The *Illuminati* has created a vast global shadow government, and their Jewish leaders secretly orchestrate all world affairs;

- Men are being born into female bodies, and women are being born into male bodies;

- Invisible "Sky Gods" will eventually rescue us from all of humanity's myriad of deadly follies;

- If you keep allowing yourself to be injected with enough mRNA CoVID-19 boosters, you will become immune to the pathogen;

- The Earth is flat and is the center of the solar system;

- The solar system has two suns, and one is merely ducking behind the other so that we can't see them at the same time;

- There exists a large portal in Antarctica where spaceships move in and out to service a vast race of miniature people that live in the hollow Earth;

- If we tune into our spiritual selves, we can raise our vibrations so high that we can walk through solid walls;

- One of my dear friends, who was a widely respected "conspiracy researcher" [he is now deceased, therefore I won't mention his name], once said during an interview on my webcast that the moon has ceased rotating around the Earth and had stopped its phases. I asked him to please repeat that statement, which he now timidly stated again. I told him very deliberately that, living in the desert 75 miles outside of Los Angeles, I would make the long drive at night several times a week during each month. One of my activities during this 90-minute drive was marveling at the starry night sky. I assured him that I witnessed the continuity of regular moon phases during these drives. There was no room for argument. He didn't argue or belabor the point. I miss my friend, but I often caught him telling some huge whoppers on talk radio shows.

Returning to the topic of The "Nature" of man, do not confuse a male of the human species with a *full-fledged Man*. A male has the potential to mature into a Man, yet it is not guaranteed. The Man that I speak of has fundamental cultural responsibilities. These characteristics have persisted across all cultures for so long that we can argue that being a Man is evolutionary. A Man naturally protects, provides, builds, accepts more rigorous workloads, aligns himself with others like himself to advance the common group interests, and is prepared to sacrifice his life to preserve the group's existence, especially when there is a challenge to the reproductive continuity of the family and group. That is a reasonable description of a Man, and then, beyond that, there is a "Man's Man."

Please, don't confuse a natural man (an adult male) with a self-declared "man" according to modern liberal societal norms.

Further, don't mistake that a natural male is necessarily a **Big Up Man.**

The corruption of nature by the industrialized environment in recent centuries has significantly impacted manhood's bio-integrity, resulting in multiple degenerate, devolutionary outcomes.

The experiences gained in a rites-of-passage program greatly distinguish a man from a male. We aim to take this further, creating men who make history – these are what we call ***Big Up Manhood***.

Just what is a Big Up Man?

A Big Up Man commands respect because he has lived an exemplary example for the community to see. He has left his mark on the broader society, and his footprints stand out clearly on multiple pathways to sovereignty and sustainable development.

A key hallmark of a Big Up Man is that his efforts have included lifting others toward their greater potential. Such a person creates those elements necessary for life's very basics. His work may include industry, creativity, science, education, security, sustenance, communication, group organizing, and leadership. Our Big Up Man example is often an employer, a healer, an author, or someone who stands out as an example of what the community recognizes as disciplined, loyal, and imaginative.

This man has considerable mechanical skills, many of which he learned in apprenticeship to those outstanding men whose generations preceded his. During his maturation, he had strong manhood models: artisans, carpenters, auto mechanics, farmers, and visible defenders of civil, social, and economic rights.

Most of us know of and can name such models of manhood that are worthy of salutation. I distinguish the Big Up Man from the typical, cliched heroes that children are programmed to call out, such as soldiers, police, doctors, lawyers, and politicians. This does not imply that individuals in such professions cannot be Big Up Men, but it requires certain tangibles such as an unshakable character, engagement with and commitment to the group, and self-sacrifice beyond the mere callings of the job.

This **Big Up Manhood** that we are focused upon comes with well-defined guidelines for morality and self-discipline, many of which I have observed over the nearly seven decades of my life. I grew up in a generation that bridged such men of high-values character to a current state of moral anarchy and widespread degeneracy. Growing up in semi-rural Ohio, it was unthinkable that a young person would utter curses in the presence of adults. The thought of cussing at one's parents or *any adult*, for that matter, was utterly out of the question. It just didn't happen. We learned much foul language during that time of youth, but you were *never* allowed to let an elder hear such words coming out of your mouth. I will never forget the day in the late 1970s on Clark Atlanta College campus when, in response to my request that a young vendor turn down his rap music because of the filthy language blaring across the plaza, he hollered, "F**k you!"

I didn't bother to respond. This new beast had risen in our community, and I was not going to invest any extra energy in engaging this mental illness. A Big Up Man knows not to risk anything of significance battling with spiritually dead *zombies* that inhabit our cities and offend our sensibilities.

Let the Dead Bury the Dead

I am at the midway point of my 38th rotation of the Sun, outside of my Mama's womb. My generation, the so-called Baby Boomers, was the bridge from the way that things were to a current state that is unsustainable to the point that our problems have become *existential*, meaning that we are at the stage of degeneration and decay that we could very well likely disappear before the next five decades have passed – fail to replicate our ethnic group within these western societies beyond 2065.

This existential challenge was the subject of my 2020 book **FADE TO BLACK: The Passing of a Great Race**. Within that book, and across numerous discussions that have followed, I intended to explain to audiences that certain fundamentals spell success for any group over the long course of time and that Afri-Amers (my reference to African Americans, Blacks, Negroes, etc.) had misplaced the core engagements that all great and historic civilizations had developed for their sustained existence. In the book, I referred to **The Six Pillars of Empire**, which I had introduced as a significant societal, economic, and sustaining set of values consistent across cultures, empires, and civilizations since the dawn of history.

Suppose a group succeeds at these **Six Pillars**. In that case, they get the opportunity to write their existence in the archives of societal development and within the grand historical archive of humanity. On the contrary, any group that fails to maintain these existential mechanisms <u>devolves into disintegration, decay, degeneration, decline, and disappearance from history</u>.

These Six Pillars of Empire are:

1) **Demographics** – People numbers matter.

2) **Resource extraction and manufacturing of finished goods** – A group must manufacture something the world needs.

3) **Intrastate trade** – A healthy group must produce the bulk of what it consumes to survive.

4) **Transnational trade** – Trading industrial surplus above the group's consumption is the only way to generate wealth.

5) **Security and expansion of territory** – As the group's numbers and businesses expand, they require more safe land for the benefit of future generations.

6) **Education of the youth to** power – Powerful groups take primary responsibility for educating young people to inherit, maintain, and expand the empire.

According to multiple analyses and honest inquiries of our scholars and Wise Elders, contemporary Afri-Amers and our cousins in other Diaspora national settings have misplaced and miserably failed at *every one* of **The Six Pillars of Empire**. Thus, without a miraculous transformation across the entire character of our ethnic conglomerate, we are doomed. We have reached the point where our group's leadership is incapable of restoring viability for the group. This crisis is much worse than these unimaginative leaders can comprehend.

It is worse than nearly all of us can even imagine. Yet, through so many conscious and unconscious processes, we are at the point of: "Let the dead bury the dead."

The "Sissification" of Generations

The "modern" man in Western societies today has too often become "punkified and sissified," as our Great Ancestor, and primary model of an Alpha Male, Khalid Abdul Muhammad, often put it. He has been converted into what he too often refers to as "his own worst enemy." This sissified male of which I speak has come under the spell of multiple manipulations. These include (but are not limited to):

- Subconscious fears from centuries of brutality, torture, and murder;

- The curse of belonging to political parties and social organizations that only use our people for what they can extract from us;

- Adopting a foreign culture that was imposed upon our group at the cracking sound of a whip or gunshot;

- Aligning our membership within supposedly empowering organizations with others' ethnic culture like posing as Greeks and Arabs;

- Become ultimately oblivious or paranoid of all avenues through which men compete for power in aggressive societies;

- He's been so humiliated by the police over the centuries that he walks down the street in a cowered *and cowardly* posture;

- He has been snitched upon, infiltrated, undermined, betrayed, and sold out by members of our ethnic community so many times that he has enculturated a fundamental mistrust of his own;

- Been castrated by the very same religion that was used as a weapon of war to neutralize the power of our indigenous cultures to preserve our people for thousands of years;

- Being told to conform to a generalized neutered position in the larger society within which our ethnicity has to function;

- Been locked out of the mainstream of social, economic, political, and respected circles within the nation;

- Come under the power of Western feminism and its undue influence on black women;

- He has had his bio-integrity corrupted by the impact of inappropriate diet and malnutrition for several generations of recent;

- So many of our members have been captured and re-enslaved by the vast medical-pharmaceutical complex that suppresses our willpower with their legal drugs;

- These same healthcare pirates, in league with powerful government agencies and industrial institutions, injected a large number of us with mRNA vaccines designed to alter our biology on various subcellular levels – they have hijacked our D.N.A. and R.N.A. functionality;

- Too many males have become fat and lazy, sluggish, disease-ridden, and incapable of defending their people against anything that demands physical strength;

- Been corrupted by a manufactured culture of self-destruction, false bravado, and pointless consumerism;

- Today's urban black male has become society's symbol of the failure of public education;

- He too often stands as a miserably failing contrast to our fathers' and grandfathers' generations, who fought will all their resources to make things better for this generation;

- His hormonal functioning was deteriorated by being born into the body of a woman who had an excess of feminizing disruptive chemicals circulating in the blood that she shared with her unborn fetus;

- He frequently consumes his favorite foods that contain high amounts of endocrine-disrupting chemicals (EDCs);

- He has been too often convinced that his sexual appetite is free-range, with no constriction on expressing unbridled lust to poke *something!*

- These last three generations of Afri-Amers have ushered more than 22.7 million of their women into abortion factories and have thus seen our national population reduced by an estimated 42 million since 1973.

- And much more has come into our immediate environment that has butchered many men's masculinity!

This modern black American has *truly* become a punkified, sissified, low-down, nasty, trifling, sorry-ass, boot-licking, shufflin', butt-scratchin', clownish Uncle Tom caricature of his former self. He has been refashioned as a new slave to his lowest nature, and the former slave master is again making a fortune off his recreation. In the words of our Dear Ancestor Del Jones, "America is a nigger factory."

Adulting is Hard?

During a recent broadcast of our Sunday morning webcast, *The Master Mind*, one of our members mentioned a theme that compelled my curiosity: "Adulting is Hard." I inquired whether this was his original reference, and he deferred to an existing dialog across social and broadcast media on the topic.

Upon researching the presence of this conversation, I realized that it had matured across multiple platforms, including books, broadcasts, the blogosphere, and onto university campuses in the form of class studies. Here is an excerpt from one such Internet blog:

> Is adulting today really more difficult than it was decades ago? Yes, it is, says Julie Lythcott-Haims, author and Stanford University's former dean of freshmen and undergraduate advising

Though some may scoff at the concerns millennials and generation Z have about adulting, Julie Lythcott-Haims, Stanford University's former dean of freshmen and undergraduate advising, says their anxieties are legitimate.

"I'm not here to quibble with the largest generation in history. I'm here to say, 'Wow, things have really changed such that this period of life you enter, if you've survived childhood, feels daunting,'" she told *The Sunday Magazine* host Piya Chattopadhyay.

Lythcott-Haims is the author of the New York Times best-seller *How to Raise an Adult*, which highlights the ways over-parenting harms children and society at large. Her new book, Your Turn: *How to Be an Adult*, builds off of her previous writing and helps readers become more comfortable with the uncertainty of adulting.[2]

There are many troubling themes within the extended CBC blog post that I wish to address. However, let me limit my critique to the following points:

- **Is adulting today really more difficult than it was decades ago?** – While the author and contributors to this sad narrative answer yes to that, from the perspective of one from the Baby Boom Generation who has borne witness to many cultural and societal changes over my seven decades of living, I don't see it this way.

- **"Yes, it is, says Julie Lythcott-Haims, author and Stanford University's former dean"** – That someone occupying a

---

[2] Adulting 101: Why being an adult is harder than ever, by Mouhamad Rachini, Canadian Broadcasting Corporation, Sunday Magazine, Jun 20, 2021

career in such a trusted institutional position, I tend to blame such individuals for the systematic weakening of the mental and psychological fortitude of younger generations. *Someone* has to take credit for this ongoing weakening of the youth. Should this woman on a college campus be beyond reproach?

- **"their anxieties are legitimate."** – While one might argue that *all* psychological stresses affecting the youth should be taken into strong consideration, I disagree from the point of view of this Big Up Man. Many of these newly appearing social anxieties result from the oversaturation of young people's lives with trifling affairs, virtual reality, liberalism, and avoidance of assuming responsibility for consequences of really poor decision-making.

- **"quibble with the largest generation"** -- The contrasts between previous generations, their existential battles for freedom, dignity, civil and human rights, and economic sustainability, can barely be compared with newer challenges for younger generations. Our "largest generation" of Baby Boomers fought against eugenicists' sterilization schemes, population control, and the breakup of the nuclear family. The generations that have followed have increasingly assumed a new moral foundation that feeds the idea of broken families, abandoned pregnancies, and avoiding responsibility for rearing the nation's children – now they complain about problems they willingly contribute to, such as the consequences of failing demographics.

- **"this period of life you enter, if you've survived childhood, feels daunting"** – I sense a strong projection of the very entitlement among these younger generations that disrupted the so-called "Me Generation" of the Baby Boomers. Yes, during my lifetime, we flipped the script that had motivated our parents and previous generations to stay focused on the fundamentals that allowed the group to survive and thrive. But, unfortunately, the big mistakes we made amplify with each subsequent generation — compounding and doubling in expansive pathological outcomes as the decades pass.

- **"over-parenting harms children and society at large"** – This notion of *over-parenting* doesn't occur in a vacuum. A spectrum of external impositions has ushered society into this shattered state of responsibility. These include: corporate profiteering from our association with toxic behaviors; failed regulation and legislation from the public sector, who are too often highly-paid agents for these pathos-exploitive non-government actors; mass media and the way it has come to be a vast social-engineering enterprise; the educational institutions that are increasingly misshaping the mental, moral, emotional, logical, and reasoning capabilities of the children that are put in their charge; and the vast liberal culture that presumes that we have the right to consent to any manner of depravity and decadence that is promoted to the general society. So, yes, "over-parenting" is problematic, but even worse is allowing all the distorted patterns of living tolerated by the dominant culture to be put on a menu for the public to consume.

- **"helps readers become more comfortable with the uncertainty of adulting"** – In my mind, NO; we don't need to become comfortable with unacceptable patterns that detract from the social behaviors that support sustainability and the conservation of our cultural integrity. Heritage is a good thing; it only comes from previous generations proving the value of intergenerational cooperation. On the contrary, we need to assist younger generations better to *become less tolerant* of ambiguity, moral liberalism, and unaccepting of pathological patterns that result in perpetual adolescence and contribute to the degeneration of the group.

I don't accept this notion that "adulting is hard" any more than the fact that many of the most valued traditions of a strong, sustainable society are not always easy to achieve. In those immortal words of the great Black orator, Frederick Douglass:

"Power concedes nothing without a demand. It never did and it never will. Find out just what any people will quietly submit to and you have found out the exact measure of injustice and wrong which will be imposed upon them, and these will continue till they are resisted with either words or blows, or with both. The limits of tyrants are prescribed by the endurance of those whom they oppress."[3]

This Book Addresses These Challenges

We could go on ad infinitum about the problems that have risen to plague our current generations. In my lifespan, I have seen these challenges come into play and actually *worsen* with each subsequent age. I try to make it clear that it was my generation of so-called Baby Boomers that turned things around after so many struggles and victories for human, civil, and economic rights, Black Power, Pan African awakening, and the restoration of all necessary to serve our group sovereignty and sustainable development.

---

[3] From the speech, West India Emancipation, by Frederick Douglass, Aug. 3, 1857, delivered at Canandaigua, New York

We are born into the most advantageous and resource-rich era of modern civilization. Yet, the data confirms that today's black community has become the epitome of dismal outlook and abysmal failure on many critical fronts. Our insanity is evident as too many of our accepted leaders continue to advocate the same tired and obsolete strategies that accompanied our disgraces over the past six decades. Analysis of the decline of our groups status between 1975 and 2022 verifies the most fatal prediction of my book, ***FADE TO BLACK: The Passing of a Great Race*** (2020) – we only have until the year 2065 until we have virtually disappeared and been replaced by the Rachel Dolezal's of society ("a former N.A.A.C.P. leader from Spokane, Washington, who made headlines in 2015 after she was exposed as a white woman who had been representing herself as black.[4]")

Big Up Manhood is being called forward to be the tip of the spear and to lead the masses toward resilience , a global outlook for our group's future, and to defend our gains and prevent another massacre of our collective destiny. Nothing less than complete victory will satisfy our call to history.

---

[4] Rachel Dolezal, White Woman Who Portrayed Herself as Black, Accused of Welfare Fraud, CNN, Fri. My 25, 2018

Where Did Our Black Manhood Go?

The Monster We Welcomed into Our Homes

Beginning in the late 1950s, a dangerous and unpredictable interloper sequestered itself in the average household. One of the great benefits of the maturity we gain over long periods is seeing the consequences of thematic changes that were initially welcomed into our lives.

Ananse Ntentan: symbol of wisdom, craftiness, creativity, and the complexities of life.

Considering what has transpired within our families since this degrading transformation began, we could not have predicted that this invited usurper would ultimately prove devastating to everyone within the home and the larger community.

The demon's seduction convinced us that this threatening intrusion was a measure of our progress – that turned out to be the first of many grievous lies it used to infect our lives. Therefore, we were reluctant to reconsider our judgments of its true value while its sinister motives undermined us all.

Our unwitting parents had worked so hard to bring us this new *cultural shape-shifting technology* – they were quite proud that they had introduced the family to this beast.

It was decades before most of us suspected that something was terribly amiss. Now, we can see the impact with more clarity. Little could we have imagined how devastating television would become to the national character sixty years ago.

I was fortunate to have grown up around the remarkable intelligence of my dad. As the years advanced and he increasingly observed the T.V.'s impact on his four sons, our father referred to our television as "the idiot box." His rebuke was ingenious.

An Analog "Virtual Reality" Stole our Mojo

Along our way, from the rise of the Black Power movement of the mid-1960s up to this current era, we have had to deal with a never-ending current of significant treachery from inside our ethnic and cultural camps. This battle has been relentless.

Across the spectrum of communications, we witnessed this infiltration of compromising cultural values that produced chasms between the generations that preceded us and our own. Into this void that appeared after the rapid transition of the civil, human, economic, and judicial rights battles of the Greatest Generation, there appeared this great interloper of television. Increasingly synthesized realities brought new marching orders for our group, to which the masses conformed. We dreamed of material goods, satiating our desires with gluttony, carnal desires, skating through life's challenges, and insatiable desires to want to be more like those who had set up apartheid conditions to corral us into subservience.

The television brought more of our households into intimate insights into the lives of whites, who turned out to be mostly fictional caricatures of an idealized society with themselves as the *apex civilization*. It wasn't real, but they, and us by default, wanted the world to believe that their television utopia was the best thing in the world, even if they had to force other societies to conform to such by the coercion of guns, bombs, and missiles. They convinced most of our trusted leaders to assist in the grand deception many believed was white supremacy.

Sellouts and Compradors Abound

Ebony Magazine online published an article in July 2012, entitled **"5 Stages of Manhood,"** which, for me, stands as the epitome of a *sorry-ass presentation* of the black man in America. Based in large part on the "Kubler-Ross "5 Stages of Grief model," it read in part:

> I spend a lot of time thinking about what it means to be a Black man in America. As circumstance would have it, I am a Black man in America, so I suppose that makes sense. However, in the wake of the killing of Trayvon Martin, I'm not alone; the rest of the country, at least temporarily, appears to be interested in the lives of Black men, particularly young Black men. Out of that tragedy has arisen the need to explain the story of Black men on a national scale.

> Of course, there isn't a single narrative, one that will definitively place all the experiences of Black men into a neat package for a curious public. However, there are commonalities, uniting factors that can help those who will never be Black men or will come into scant contact with Black men to get a general sense of what shapes the lives of Black men. There's the hope that, perhaps, the more the world knows about us, the fewer Trayvons there will be. A prayer set out into the darkness, no doubt, but that in itself is a part of the Black male experience.

The **"5 Stages of Black Manhood"** detailed by the *Ebony* article's author Mychal Denzel Smith, follow with a few excerpted lines defining the author's introspect:

1. **Denial** – "...eventually something pushes a previously dormant voice in the mind of every Black man to say "wake up, you're Black" and he doesn't want to believe it. This isn't so much about the denial of one's Blackness as it is a denial about world's reaction to that Blackness. No one wants to believe their mere existence is a problem..."

2. **Anger** – "You're born into a legacy that includes slavery, lynching, Jim Crow, marches, protests, and riots. From the moment you're old enough to know what it is, you're told that it's likely you'll end up in prison, and you start to believe it... Black male anger isn't an anomaly, it's a consequence of breathing."

3. **Bargaining** – "A large part of being a Black man is understanding that you can't tell all of the truth, or you won't be alive long enough to tell any truth at all... This is where you find the acceptance of reductive histories of Black male heroes, chopping their legacies down to near meaningless platitudes like "I Have a Dream" or "By Any Means Necessary"... It's wanting the world to take in the genius of James Baldwin so badly, that you agree in principle to never mention the fact of his sexuality, or even come to hate that part of him yourself. It's not even bothering to learn Bayard Rustin's name."

4. **Depression** – "...When it is assumed that Black men are on rampant drug users and alcoholics, one wouldn't view that behavior as a sign of anything more than their natural state... Depression is the inevitable consequence of every day facing

a society that makes it clear it doesn't believe you have a right to exist."

5. **Acceptance** – "What it does mean is that Black men are consistently remembering that they are Black men, and that means something wicked for the rest of the world.…It's the embracing of one's Black self, gay self, bisexual self, and/or trans self as one whole. This is about creating culture that becomes indispensable [sic]."

I find it both sad and outrageous that the Afri-Amer community has for so long regarded *Ebony Magazine* (E.M.) as cutting-edge journalism intended to present an empowering voice to our people.   Thinking back to all the E.M. issues that I've encountered in my life, I now consider it to be worthless – *except* for the February 1987 issue featuring the Bachelors of the Year, of which my twin brother and I were selected for the photo essay!

E.M. has always been elitist, supporting the *cult of personality*, which has been the most ineffective style of leadership, and has sacrificed the self-esteem of Black Womanhood for a pittance of compensation from its corporate advertisers.

In *direct contrast* to the list of 5 Stages of Black Manhood put forward by the compradors at *Ebony*, I put forward these as serving as foundation for a truly redemptive and resilient pathway:

The 5 Stages of Big Up Manhood

1. **Consciously Aware** – A lifetime of experiences shapes our subconscious mind landscape. For a boy to grow up in a home where is masculine values are shaped in large part by stability, mutually-supportive partnership between the

parents, and an abundance of creative talent, encourages that child to seek reflection and validation of these positive attributes in the larger world as the boy grows into subsequent stages of manhood.

2. **Emotionally Stable** – One of the common characteristics to be found in the mature, socially-adapted adult is the ability to summon the values of logic and reason as means of survival and traversing society and the world. Emotions are an essential part of our human nature. However, out of control, emotions are acidic and can lead to injury and destruction to those things regarded as valuable to the individual and the group.

3. **Uncompromising** – I frequently admonish my students to "set and get your goals." Planning one's key life expressions, such as education, career, artistic engagements, building a family, and graceful aging are all wonderful examples of where we should not compromise on those aspects of the life plan that we firmly commit to achieving. Don't let nobody sway you from those things that you have decided are essential to your well-being.

4. **Motivated** – Where our passions, emotions, commitments of time and resources are best invested is largely determined by primary motivation. Within this ***Big Up Manhood*** cultural model, we frequently emphasize the critical need to have a *massive transformative purpose* (MTP) that moves us through the world and guides our life journeys. With the right MTP in place, one will never be burdened by procrastination and lack of creative imagination.

5. **Resilient** – No matter what comes along as obstacles or setbacks to our visions and dreams of the future we would

create for our generations, we must, above all, bounce back from adversity and persist toward our most cherished destinations. The late great Jamaican reggae artist Peter Tosh expressed how he showed resilience against life's setbacks. Tosh sang:

"I'm Sittin' in the midday sun and wondering
Where my meal's coming from.
After working so hard,
Not even a piece of bread at the yard.
I really try, try, try, but I got to
Pick myself up, dust myself off.
Start all over again."

What Happened to the Black Revolution?

The following is excerpted from my 1999 book ***THE ROAD TO POWER Seven Steps to an African Global Order***:

We have analyzed our greatest recent failures to secure visions of empowerment. As we move forward in a rapid fashion we must be mindful not to repeat some of our most reckless errors during similar past endeavors—there are those who will resist us and they can be expected to be very serious about their opposition.

Was it even clear within our minds what a Black Revolution was even about? Often we recall those profound lyrics of funk-jazz poet Gil Scott Heron, "The Revolution will not be televised." You could make the argument that nearly everything the entertainment media aims at our youth has been anti-revolutionary, and that assumption would be hard to contest. Maybe my memory is failing me, but I don't believe that there ever was a clear consensus on what "The Revolution" was going to entail anyway.

There was no plebiscite, no election, not even a Gallop or CNN poll, to determine what would be the primary goals of the Black Revolution. Some groups tried hard to define it. The Panthers had a ten-point platform of action. The Nation of Islam had a similar set of principles, but the great majority of the so-called 'Colored/Negro/Black/Nigga/Afro-American/African-American/ African population couldn't get along with either one of those two groups long enough to even examine their programs and give a thumbs up or a thumbs down; we still can't even all agree upon what to call ourselves!

We were not prepared for a long-term struggle. The 1960s and 1970s constituted a significant era in the U.S., a critical moment in history. Yet, most people were detached bystanders to the major historical events; or passive/active participants in a grand theater to which they were mostly oblivious. What we didn't know at the time was that the greatest revolution, the theft of mass identity by an intoxicating entertainment media, was occurring right before our eyes as we tuned in to the new national pastime, most days from after school until late at night.

What was needed was brilliant analysts, like Malcolm. He could articulate to the masses that history would be made tomorrow, this week, before the year was out, and that **we had better get mobilized and become**

participants in it. And as the 1970s wore on, the newly discovered indulgences of affluence, access, sensuality, and chemical retreat further blinded many youth's vision. Revolutionary visions degraded into hazy dreams confounded by reefer, soda-flavored wine, some crazy psychedelics that white boys were selling, and the most addictive and deadly drug of the century—television.

Television kicked our black Umoja butts. We couldn't tell where we came from and didn't have a clue about where we were going. But we sure got to know a lot of people along the way—virtual people, that is. There were virtual lovers, virtual gangsters, virtual secret agents, virtual saints, virtual vixens, virtual superheroes, virtual bandits, virtual athletes, virtual foreigners, virtual preachers, *more* virtual preachers, virtual feminists, virtual enemies, virtual role models, virtual junkies, virtual failures, virtual shootings, virtual murders, virtual food—real depression, real apathy, and real defeat.

That's what happened to the Black Revolution.

Our Global Fight Against Apartheid

There is a historical narrative referred to as the "civil rights movement" that is shared across national borders, languages, and distinct cultural communities across communities of Africans on the Mother Continent and across the Diaspora.

The online dictionary Merriam Webster categorizes "apartheid" as a synonym of racial segregation, yet we know it was much more. As well, those of us that are astute students of history know that racism in America, which included our parallel version of apartheid which is called "Jim Crow," was far harsher than merely keeping ethnic nationalities separate.

This American apartheid system included every description of crimes against humanity, spanning separatism, caste-based hierarchy, violent suppression, the near-slave condition of peonage that we called sharecropping, lynching, mass murder, child rape, kidnapping, torture, wage slavery, chain-gangs, land theft, eugenics, mass sterilization, promoting abortion, medical experimentation, imposition of false religions, state-sponsored terrorism, collective punishment, prison camps, extensive surveillance, denial of basic human rights, widespread starvation, mass killings of enlisted soldiers, the use of weapons of mass destruction against our members including biowarfare, chemical, and toxin agents, nuclear radiation, murdering parents in front of their children and children in front of their parents, along with most every other description of genocidal barbarism that one could describe.

And still we rose. We rose from the dead level of being deprived of every aspect of a free human's life and dignity. These beastly colonizing forces assaulted us all over the world, stole our resources including labor, and enriched themselves while all the while condemning us as lowly good-for-nothings. Under the worst of their apartheid living conditions our ancestors still found many ways to express their humanity — even creating music that expressed our woeful condition that also served to restore our dignity, if nothing more than to facilitate greater tolerance of our burdens of misery.

And still we rose, and today, still we rise. We will rise tomorrow with the dawn. And days after that... and seasons, years, decades and centuries until the very end of human time. We are Africans and we are Rising.

We have risen countless mornings to fight numerous apartheid frontlines that we found on every continent except for Antarctica. We fought against all the major empires across history, from the Persians to the Anglos. We have sacrificed much to stand against the brutalities of genocidal apartheid. If needed, we must and we will stand in this generation as well.

We do not fight because we have a blood lust for war, cultural plunder, and pillaging of the wealth of weaker people. We fight because our culture, spiritual nature, traditions, perspective of history, morality and logical reasoning dictates that we fight in this generation so that those who follow ours will have a better chance to make the lives for themselves and their families they truly deserve.

As Big Up Men, we will fight and die if it is necessary to preserve our unbroken heritage. As **Big Up Manhood**, we must prepare our sons to fight even at greater levels when they reach the age of responsible manhood. This is our sacred inheritance, and we cannot violate the sanctity of our Great Ancestors' sacrifices. We WILL fight, if necessary, to preserve life.

Seeing the American civil rights struggle in context

One of the wonderful aspects of becoming an Elder in society is that your life has mirrored many important societal transformations. Born in 1955, I have been alive through so many major occurrences and changes in the world. A few of the most significant and impactful changes during my years include, but are *not* limited to:

- The finalizing of the domestic fight against American apartheid and gaining of increased civil and economic rights;

- The signing of national legislation intended to ensure universal access to civil and voting rights;

- The offering of Affirmative Action programs to Blacks that ended up being usurped by newly-declared "minorities";

- The rise of an urban black middle class;

- The global impact of the Cold War East-West hostilities;

- The 1963 assassination, a de facto coup d' état in the U.S.;

- A series of government-sponsored murders against civil and human rights leaders, political figures, and influential celebrities;

- The rise of the Black Power Movement and its suppression;

- Waves of cultural shifts prompted by electronic entertainment, mass media, and social engineering;

- A broad-based degeneration of family, morality, and business integrity;

- Pan-African anti-colonial liberation battles and resistance;

- Impactful social movements involving feminism, homosexuality, hippies, consumerism, narcissism, corporatism, and the decline of organized religions;

- A shift from Negroes, to Blacks, to African-Americans, to Africans;

- The space race era and the change from transistor to printed circuit electronics have come to dominate our lives;

- A rise to dominance by the profit-driven international medical-pharmaceutical complex;

- Introduction of computers across society and the spread of personal computers, along with the birth and sovereignty of the Internet;

- The U.S. begins to decline from the apex of its global empire;

- At the turn of the 21st Century, phenomena like the Asian Tigers, Africa Rising, population growth in the global south, the demographic decline among Europeans and rich Asians;

- And hundreds of other significant changes just in my life.

Beyond question, these last seven decades have brought some of the most monumental and rapid changes to our world. Even the notion that our fate is intertwined with eight billion other humans is often too amazing to consider.

We are often cast into a state of overwhelm at the pace and volume of major changes coming at us. There can be no denial that the speed of these significant changes is increasing with each passing year, decade, or generation. Just as were our parents and previous generations, we must realize that it is our time to confront the major and minor challenges to family, community, society, nations, and humanity.

Malcolm X, Amos Wilson, and John Henrick Clarke are three of our favorite futurists that, from an African-centered perspective, instructed us on how to read these societal changes in real-time and, from that position, analyze, forecast, and empower our group interests accordingly. But have we really paid heed to the instructions of these wise and esteemed scholars for our people's destiny?

We Passed the Torch, Only to See It Snatched Away

Previously, I noted a list of significant societal changes during my lifespan. This partial accounting certainly includes the passing of the empowerment struggle to the Black Power movement. From the perspective of this **Big Up Manhood** focus, these transferences of power from one generation to the next are key to our existence. As this process proceeds across the entirety of one or more centuries, then we not only have societal continuity, but we can thus develop civilization growth and rise to higher levels of sustainable development. Long-term productivity and viability are the roots of the *evolution of civilizations*.

Among many major setbacks that have happened to our people along this long Maafa Journey of capture, enslavement, emancipation, and many decades of violent humiliation, we have frequently confronted government-sponsored violence as an extension of societal oppression.

One such ugly chapter of American history was the Federal Bureau of Investigation's notorious *counter-intelligence program* (COINTELPRO) and the wars against black militancy, the American Indian Movement, radical left anti-war protesters, and the Chicano movement.

Although the discovery of "The COINTELPRO Papers" led to the official shutdown of COINTELPRO after 1971, we know that similar programs, underway at that time, escaped scrutiny and functioned into the 1990s and beyond; I documented this in my 1997 book **RAP, HIP HOP & THE NEW WORLD ORDER.** Two programs I highlighted in the book were:

[A] modern version of COINTELPRO, most likely encoded in the FBI's TOPLEV BLACPRO acronym, has targeted the hip-hop generation for similar counterintelligence measures. The existence of the TOPLEV and a similar COMTEL program was the subject of one of our favorite research journals, Covert Action Information Bulletin (CAIB, since renamed Covert Action Quarterly).

I then went on to cite two paragraphs from CAIB, showcasing their superb work at investigative reporting on these controversial and disturbing developments:

Officially, the FBI's so-called Counterintelligence Program (COINTELPRO) was ended by the Bureau in 1971. The New York Times quoted a former FBI official involved in COINTELPRO that the program was continuing apace at least as of the time he left the Bureau in mid-1974.

In 1979, CAIB received information from a knowledgeable source that COINTELPRO was continuing. Further, it was then operating in Puerto Rico and elsewhere under two new FBI cryptonyms: COMTEL and TOPLEV, presumably for Communications Intelligence and Top Level... 1fIndeed, there is documented evidence in the Church Committee report of TOPLEVs existence. The FBI alerted its field offices in October 1967 that it was initiating a program for "the development of ghetto-type racial informants," and that it was expanding its operative "Black Nationalist Groups TOPLEV Informant Program."[5]

I highlight this sordid history to keep a spirit of resistance alive from one generation to another. There will be resistance and

---

[5] Cited in CONSPIRACIES AND HIGH CRIMES, by Keidi Awadu, 1998 pgs. 44-45

pushback from entrenched forces that see our liberation and ascendence as a threat to their hegemonic position that they have achieved by plundering weaker societies for centuries, even millennia. Things change, yet too often, they remain the same. Our critical need for vigilance is within the flame passed from generation to generation if we are to remain great people, rising to our full potential for this 21st Century and beyond.

Big Up Man, see yourself on the frontlines of this intergenerational contest for liberty, equality, and brotherhood. You know that the world is changing at an ever-more-rapid pace. You instinctively know that you must engage with your natural talents and abilities. You can make a difference. Big Up Man, rise and take your stance today and for all time.

A Collapse of Black Manhood

"It is criminal to teach a man not to defend himself when he is the constant victim of brutal attacks." – Malcolm X

I began writing this book midway through America's Black History Month commemoration. By now, most of us have had an opportunity to understand the roots of this celebration with the significant contribution of Dr. Carter G. Woodson's efforts to restore a sense of historical perspective and cultural pride to people of African ancestry in the U.S. It is imperative that our children and future generations would inherit and preserve this proud legacy that Dr. Woodson highlighted.

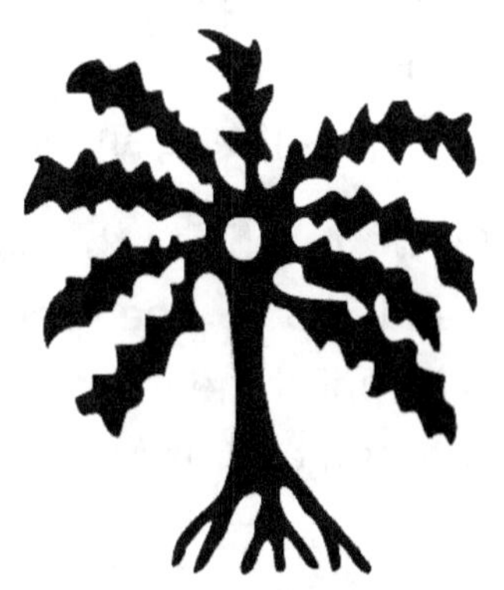

Abe Dua: wealth, resourcefulness, and self-sufficiency

Over the years, via my 20-year legacy of webcast radio, I made it a point to expand our historical acclamations to a global perspective. Black history is more than American history. Black history is *world history*, therefore, we might best refer to this renaissance of a self-determined *global narrative* as **African world history**. Our story includes various Diaspora communities in North, Central, and South Americas and across the C.A.R.I.C.O.M. island nations.

Our long Songhai Journey spans the European, Asian, and Australian continents. We acknowledge that this global African family has spread its branches across the Pacific Ocean archipelagos. We ARE a global people with an estimated 1.725 billion people of African Ancestry worldwide. Our heart is the African mother continent. As we realize an even greater potential, approaching 2.5 billion by the year 2050, we soon realize the true meaning of **"Africa Rising – WE got next!"**

Yet our long history of enduring many existential problems has faced many challenges along this course. It serves best to acknowledge our transformation over the past century of global struggle. By confronting and overcoming what Malcolm X referred to as "brutal attacks" that challenged our survival, we come to know who we truly are and what would be a triumphant fate and ideal destiny for our noble race.

As we reach for the stars, we must always remember that we stand upon the shoulders of Giants. Let's review the accomplishments and challenges that have challenged the various generations.

The Greatest Generation

- The Greatest Generation was born between 1901-1927
- They experienced The Great Migration from southern states
- Their contributed Black labor saved the nation during WWII
- Supplied as the backbone for the nation's agricultural labor force
- Established a primary post-war position within the urban workforce, occupying prime real estate in U.S. cities
- Their hegemonic position within the urban landscape downshifted rapidly in the 1960s and early 1970s
- They began to expand our national and cultural identities to an empowering of a Pan-African consciousness

The Baby Boomers

- The Baby Boomers were born between 1946-1964

- Inherited the strongest economic position for the black family since emancipation

- Benefited from living within a wealthy superpower nation with greater access to education, middle-class families, nutrition, healthcare, and employment opportunities

- Due to the shocks of the 1960s, Boomers became a traumatized, psyche-damaged generation that fell victim to a complex eugenics plot and adopted many degenerate habits

- Bought into media-generated character models and lifestyles that ultimately proved debilitating

- Squandered the valuation of black labor as a factor in defining the wealth of family, community, and the nation

- Adopted a broad set of poor health habits that fueled the increase of epidemics of preventable chronic diseases

- Established a persisting trend of giving birth to a generation weaker than that of its parents

Generation X

- Generation X's birth years were between 1965-1980

- They continued to feed the newly established patterns of degeneration and decay;

- Reduced our group's total fertility rate (TFR) to below replacement;

- Established the doubling of rates of alternative sex lifestyles, which has continued with subsequent generations, and escalated the *sissification* (feminization) of the males;

- Has increased the commonality of interracial childbirths;

- Increased the excessive rate of black children born out of a married two-parent household, currently reported at 70.1% [6]

- According to a January 2023 CDC Vital Statistics report, for the years 2020-2021, while the general fertility rate for "Hispanic" women rose 1%, and non-Hispanic White women rose 3%, it *declined* during that time for non-Hispanic Black women by 3% and 2% for Asian women;

- According to Vital Statistics, "The U.S. TFR has generally been below replacement since 1971 and has consistently been below replacement since 2008. Total Fertility Rates were below replacement for all race and Hispanic-origin groups in 2021, except for non-Hispanic NHOPI (Native Hawaiians Other Pacific Islanders) women."

- From 2016-2021, Black women's lifetime fertility declined from 1.832 to 1.625. The replacement rate is 2.1 childbirths;

- The intrusion of white feminist values into black family affairs has disrupted nearly every aspect of family, including the lifelong incidence of marriage, unmarried childbirths, spinsterhood, age at first childbirth, total fertility, and homosexuality – all of these conditions are worsening with each generation;

---

[6] Births to unmarried women, National Vital Statistics Reports Volume 72, No. 1, January 21, 2023, CDC Vital Statistics

- Gen X established a decline in literacy and educational achievement, which is more prominent among young males;

- We see a shocking rise in metabolic disorders and non-communicable diseases impacting younger generations.

Generation Why Care Anymore?

As I write today, another mass shooting in the U.S. has captured news headlines. Checking with an authoritative website that tracks this carnage, yesterday's mass shooting at Michigan State University in East Lansing, which killed four and injured another five before the gunman killed himself, brings the 2023 tally of American mass shootings to 73 and counting. This slaughter occurred in the first 44 days of the new calendar year. Something is terribly wrong here.[7] There were seven reported mass shootings on January 1st, 2023, alone.

Surely there are limitations to what a **Big Up Manhood** can do to put an end to this mass murder that is occurring within this nation and disproportionately impacting our urban communities. We must consider the necessary security measures that increase safety and mental health stability among our younger generations. We are again existentially challenged on multiple fronts. As a manner of *demographic triage*, we are forced to prioritize the self-protection systems within our capacity. We must also do this while in such a damaged state due to our long struggle for survival.

---

[7] List of mass shootings in the United States in 2023, Wikipedia, citing Gun Violence Archive, Feb. 14, 2023

Generation Y: The Millennials Dominate

We have talked about the transformation of our ethnic group between the generations.

The Millennials, aka Generation Y, were born between 1981 and 1996, making them between 27 and 42 years old. With a population estimated at 75 million in the U.S., this is the largest demographic bubble after the Baby Boomers. The Washington DC public policy organization *Brookings Institution's* research writer William H. Frey January referred to this group as a "demographic bridge to America's diverse future."[8]

> The millennial generation, over 75 million strong is America's largest — eclipsing the current size of the postwar baby boom generation. Millennials make up nearly a quarter of the total U.S. population, 30 percent of the voting age population, and almost two-fifths of the working age population.

> Most notably, the millennial generation, now 44 percent minority, is the most diverse adult generation in American history. While its legacy is yet to be determined, this generation is set to serve as a social, economic, and political bridge to chronologically successive (and increasingly) racially diverse generations.

> As the cultural generation gap graphic shows, while both the post-millennial and pre-millennial populations were majority white in 2015 (51.5 percent and 68.4 percent, respectively), both population groups are projected to

---

[8] The millennial generation: A demographic bridge to America's diverse future, by William H. Frey, Brookings Institution, January, 2018

substantially decrease their shares of the white population by 2035, to 46 percent and 64.8 percent, respectively. Yet, even in 2035, the millennial generation will represent a bridge to the more racially diverse young adult population.

Demographics have long stood to gauge the measure of any group's impact on society, nations, and the evolution of civilizations. Regarding Gen Y, certain characteristics have firmly differentiated the Millennials from all previous generations. These are especially apparent regarding institutional decline as we measure family, marriage, and childbirthing. Returning to the *Brookings'* research:

Millennials are slower than earlier generations to get married, have children, and leave their parents' homes. The median age of marriage was lowest during the 1950s—at age 20 for women and 22 for men. By 2015, these rose to ages 27 and 29, respectively. Allowing longer periods for higher education and rising women's labor force participation have pushed up the ages of marriage and childbearing over the decades. However, the Great Recession and resulting housing crash led millennials to even further delay these domestic milestones.

The broad pattern toward delay in marriage has been followed by millennials in each racial and ethnic group. **Blacks continue to exhibit the lowest share of persons who are currently married—halving their share, at ages 25-34, from 47 percent in 1980 to 23 percent.** Just as with the national patterns, long term shifts toward later

> marriage have been amplified for all groups by recent economic conditions. [Emphasis added]

I would add that, at a total fertility rate that measured 1.625 childbirths to mostly Millennials, this is the lowest rate for black women in the U.S. in recorded history. These numbers are similar for our fellow diaspora cousins in places like the UK and Canada, although they diverge based on the country of origin.

According to the British Office of National Statistics, the TFR for the United Kingdom as a whole was 1.65 in 2019, which is below the replacement level of 2.1. Here are the TFRs for some of the largest ethnic groups in the UK:

- White British: 1.59
- Indian: 1.65
- Pakistani: 2.92
- Bangladeshi: 2.13
- Black African: 2.36
- Black Caribbean: 1.76
- Chinese: 1.49

According to Statistics Canada, the national TFR in Canada was 1.39 in 2020, which is below the replacement level of 2.1. Here are the projected TFRs for various ethnic groups in Canada:

- White: 1.42
- South Asian: 1.87
- Chinese: 1.34
- Black: 2.03
- Filipino: 2.21
- Latin American: 1.78
- Arab: 2.12

From the Brooking Institution's revealing research report and multiple other sources, we share key characteristics of the Millennials' impact on society beyond their demographic data.

- Although the Millennials are now in their early 40s, they are still synonymous with youthfulness;

- They have attained higher levels of education than previous gens and, subsequently, have higher income levels. A third of Millennials achieved a college education by 2015, compared to less than 30% in 2000 and about 25% in 1980;

- They are born into a highly technological age, as well as having the experience of 9/11 and its aftermath as a powerful impact on their world outlook;

- An estimated 80% of the group's members live within a 100-mile radius of their childhood home;

- Migrating Millennials have relocated to major cities such as L.A., New York, and Washington, DC;

- They are noted as an adaptive and creative generation;

- Thanks to their technical abilities and creative adaptability, they can be quite astute in their careers and task-oriented instead of merely focusing on time.

As well there are several criticisms of Millennials' behavioral tendencies. These include:

- They have been accused of not understanding "the difference between being an entrepreneur and doing something entrepreneurial."

- Some perceive that their natural tech savvy makes them overly confident, pretentious about their expertise, and pushy;

- They are sometimes criticized as unfocused and constantly distracted;

- The type of collaboration that is a hallmark of teamwork and leadership seems to not be a high quality of this generation;

- Millennials don't like to answer telephone calls or to initiate them, preferring to text than talk, something that irks older generations;

- They are noted for an inability to give or take criticism and overly sensitive to their feelings.

- They are accused of talking more than listening and sometimes coming off as "acting too cool to care.";

- Too much multitasking and unwilling to take the time to learn unfamiliar tasks or business models.

I am reluctant to heap an excess of fault on younger generations; after all, they are "products of the product." Each younger generation reflects those that preceded it. Still, we must have accountability for each member of society, no matter their age categorization. Certain things are just right, reflect intelligence, and are vital to a group's integrity and survival.

This chapter has been about the decline of manhood over the past century and the consequences that this spells for families, communities, ethnic groups, nations, and whole civilizations. Yet, because of this generalized focus, we cannot let up on whatever criticism must be meted out toward corrective practices that lead to sustainability and prosperity for the larger group.

Ultimately, competence becomes the highest priority for developing leadership for the collective. As Big Up Men, we must comprehend what is happening in the world that we live in and the world that we intend to create for our children's and future generations' benefits.

A Big Up Man Should Be Able To...

"When you can do the common things of life in an uncommon way, you will command the attention of the world." – George Washington Carver

"Someone's sitting in the shade today because someone planted a tree a long time ago."
– Warren Buffett

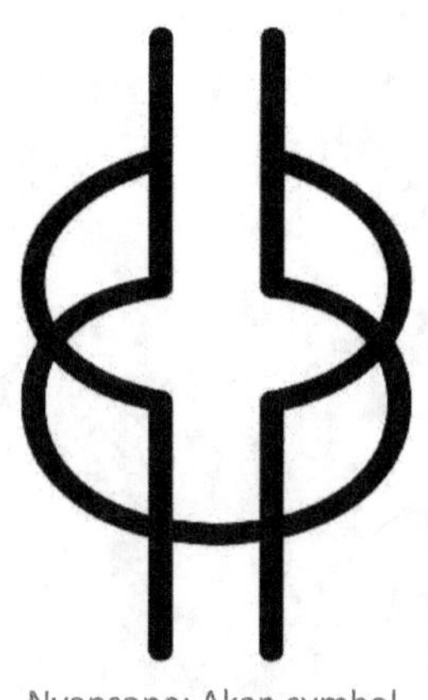
Nyansapo: Akan symbol of wise leadership, ingenuity & Intelligence

As **Big Up Men**, we must raise the standards by which we identify as individuals and the community duties, roles, and responsibilities expected of our members. A proverb from the ancient Nile Valley civilization of Kemet states, "An uninitiated male is still a child."

As the Elder guiding this rites-of-passage program and initiation into what we call the **Big Up Manhood**, I've brought forward a broad set of guidelines and standards for our members to use as a baseline for behaviors that confirm our transformation.

I ask only of the initiates what I require of myself; there shall be no hypocrisy or impossible standards being pushed herein.

What we are firmly doing is seeking to project a new leadership standard, to generate a reliable generation of men that are committed to sustainable development, and to project ourselves as *the tip of the spear* that plunges into the heart of all who would rise to oppose our freedom, dignity, and sovereign advancement.

The world needs this type of leader to rise, and we stand strong to heed this sacred call.

- Do at least 40 push-ups without hesitation; a Big Up Man has prepared his body to respond to emergencies requiring strength.

- Engage in fasting for a minimum of 3 days straight on water only.

- Contain his emotions until the primary problem is solved.

- Stop eating foods that undermine his masculinity, cold turkey (pun intended)!

- Read at least 3-4 books a year, and enroll and actively engage in book study circles.

- Teach valuable work craftsmanship to the younger generation (i.e., woodworking, auto mechanics, plumbing, carpentry, gardening, music, tailoring, etc.)

- Cooperate and collaborate with others toward fulfilling collective actions that uplift and sustain the family and community.

- Suppress his ego and recognize when someone attempts to impart wisdom to him and others (shut up and learn).

- Make a wealth development plan for his family and children to thrive optimally and stick to that plan without unwarranted deviation.

- Be loyal and true to his interpersonal commitments.

- Refrain from selling his labors to those that ruthlessly exploit, undermine, and abuse the economics of the family, community, and larger societies.

- Actively and adequately resist and repel the "sissification" of the males in his generation and those to follow.

- Exercise his right to openly express his inner truths and respect others who express their right to free speech.

- Bond with others in a Sacred Brotherhood of mutual support.

- Demonstrate his prime interest and commitment to an MTP (*Massive Transformative Purpose*).

- Write a clear statement of purpose, a creed he pledges daily to live by.

- Not allow his life mission to be emotionally reactive and dictated by forces outside his control spectrum. Common "isms" (doctrines) that affect the bulk of society do not necessarily deter the self-determined man from making the world work for his ultimate benefit.

Consolidating Biological Integrity

"The Great Culling of the human race already has begun. It is being done through chemicals added to our drinking water, food, medicines, and the air we breathe - chemicals that have the known effect of reducing fertility and shortening lifespan." – G. Edward Griffin

Living Superfood Research

Food is Nature's most perfect medicine – If you have been following my research, writings, broadcasts, and other public communications, you have heard this statement many times. It is true. This sentiment has been expressed for more than 2000 years. The Greek physician Hippocrates, himself a student of Imhotep through the Temple of Asclepius (the Greek name for Imhotep), is credited with the famous quote, "Let your food be your medicine, and your medicine be your food."

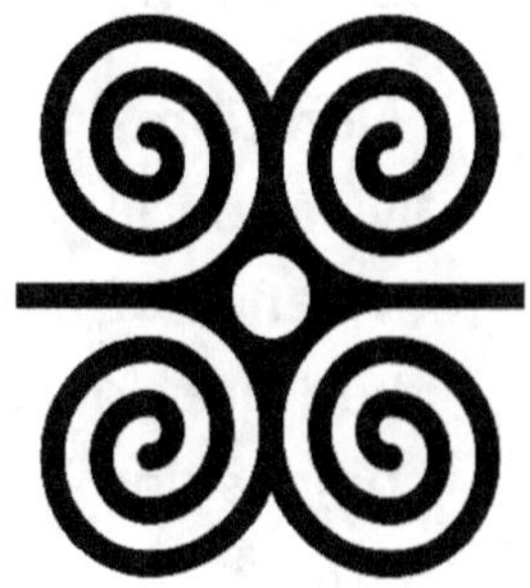

Dwennimmen, the Ram's Horns. symbol of humility together with Strength.

Another statement attributed to the famous Greek healing scholar is one of my favorite quotes: "Leave your drugs in the chemist's pot if you can heal the patient with food."

Many natural health advocates, and increasingly over the past century, have proven the practicality of choosing nutrition as our preferred healing system. It is also profoundly true that as this natural pathway reverses disease and disorder, it will prevent these pathologies from becoming established within our bodies.

I have served my community as a clinical nutritionist consultant for a dozen years. I developed a system called *Living Superfood* that has *full-spectrum hyper-nutrition* at its core. This full spectrum encompasses the complete range of eight critical classes of nutrients that are required to sustain optimal human health. These essential nutrients are at the core of my clinical nutrition comprehension as they are centric to my regimen of optimal health, high performance, and a healthy lifespan.

The eight classes of critical nutrients are water, vitamins, minerals, protein, carbohydrates, essential fatty acids, enzymes, and fiber. In the book **LIVING SUPERFOOD RESEARCH: Don't Get Sick, Stay Off Drugs, and Live a Long Time**, I explored these eight critical nutrients in depth. Briefly, let's review each:

1. **Hydration / Water** – "Water is Life" for humans and every living species. When scientists search the cosmos looking for evidence of planets that could support life, it is water that they are looking for. Ideally, 70 percent of our body composition is hydration, just as is 70 percent of the Earth's surface.

2. **Vitamins** – These organic molecules are essential for all aspects of functioning for species. For the most part, vitamins are not synthesized by the human body and must be obtained through nutrition.

3. **Minerals** – Like vitamins, minerals are critically needed to support every aspect of living organisms. Our body requires eight major minerals and nearly a hundred more *microminerals* to sustain optimal health.

4. **Proteins (Amino Acids)** – Cells comprise the basic units within our bodies that constitute life; cells combine to make

tissues that form organs and organic systems. In turn, cells are made up of molecules, which are present in numbers so great that their numbers are virtually indescribable. Specialized organs manufacture these molecules within the body from raw materials known as amino acids. Our diet requires a spectrum of 22 such amino acids for optimal function. These amino acids are derived from the proteins that serve as nutrition.

5. **Carbohydrates** – In chemistry, a carbohydrate is a biomolecule made from carbon, hydrogen, and oxygen. In nutrition, carbs are simple sugar molecules that are our energy source through the formation of glucose, glycogen, and fat cells (adipose tissues). Carbs are a critical and necessary part of healthy nutrition in their natural form as polysaccharides. However, overly processed and refined, such as the case of white sugar, white flour, and high-fructose corn syrup, these substances become increasingly toxic the more they are consumed.

6. **Essential fatty acids (EFAs)** – EFAs are critically important across all bodily functions, from the cells' structures to bio-integrity across all the body's 17 functional systems. However, these are not synthesized by the body (although the body uses EFAs to manufacture other needed micro chemicals); therefore, we must obtain fatty acids from our diet.

7. **Enzymes** – These are naturally occurring chemicals that serve as catalytic agents to make chemical reactions occur within the body. While not much in the attention of the food-consuming public, enzymes are critically important to every aspect of metabolism, the mechanics of living systems.

8. **Fiber** – Made of carbohydrates, fiber is the part of carbohydrate molecules that is not broken down during digestion into simple sugars for fuel. Two forms of fiber are soluble and insoluble. They aid in detoxing the blood and digestive system and feed the functioning of the 100 trillion healthy bacteria that are essential life partners inhabiting the gut.

Ideally, we would formulate our daily nutrition centered around these eight critical nutrients. It would be best to consume them in their full spectrum through fresh, organic, locally-sourced fruits, vegetables, roots, nuts and seeds, and whole grains.

Aiming toward the highest integrity of our nutrition, we would avoid consuming foodstuffs that contain this spectrum of nutrients but are unfortunately contaminated by substances that undermine optimal nutrition. These toxic foods include meat, dairy, eggs, highly processed foods, refined grains, and chemicals masquerading as food. Much of these compromising foods comprise the Standard American Diet, often called the acronym S.A.D. diet.

In ***LIVING SUPERFOOD RESEARCH,*** I supplied a list of modern eating styles, grading them from *the worst* to the *best of the best*. In brief, this 11-level hierarchy consisted of the following:

1. Junk food

2. Fast food (including most restaurants)

3. Standard American Diet (S.A.D.)

4. Modified SAD

5. Vegetarian

6. Vegan

7. 80/20 Vegan (80% raw, 20% cooked)

8. Raw Vegan

9. Vegan with detoxification

10. Living Superfood

11. Orthomolecular medicine

I believe that the **Big Up Man** must completely comprehend these issues of optimized nutrition and raising oneself high on this hierarchy of eating styles to activate the immense potential of his biological functioning fully. However, on the contrary, eating low on this categorization of best nutrition is to commit oneself to a life at great risk of disruption by acute and chronic diseases and disorders. Therefore, it is our choice to live within the premise that "Food is Nature's most perfect medicine."

Moving your diet to the top of the eating style hierarchy is one of the smartest moves you could make toward activating your ***Big Up Manhood*** lifestyle to its greatest potential. As one man who made a powerful impact on world history stated: "Nothing will benefit human health and increase the chances for survival of life on Earth as much as the evolution to a vegetarian diet." – *Albert Einstein*.

Furiously Vegan: 21 Steps to Restore Youthful Vitality

The following is excerpted from the introduction to my 2021 book ***FURIOUSLY VEGAN***.

Sometimes I wonder if people might get annoyed at my too-frequent boasts about being "the healthiest senior citizen in the world," the tangibility of which is just too powerful for me to suppress. I LOVE being healthy, vital, youthful-looking, and vibrantly energetic. I greatly appreciate that I have been graced with a sharp mind, to the point that when introduced by some of the learned broadcasters of our generation, it is almost embarrassing when they rave over the diversity of functional accomplishments that I bring to the conversation.

I remember those inspiring lyrics Donny Hathaway sang from his seminal song: "To be young, gifted and black. That's where it's at."

I claim that mantel. I AM young. I AM gifted, and I AM proud to be black. In fact, a greeting that I often share when someone asks me, "how are you doing?" My frequent response is, "We black and we shine."

Many people are motivated by the abundance of Life. Unfortunately, too many seem excited primarily by scarcity, pain, fear, anxieties regarding the future, and demonstrable anger because they feel they are getting left behind. In contrast, others prosper at the victim's expense. We each can see the proverbial "cup as half-empty or half-full." We just need to be assured that it is our *conscious decision* to express optimism or pessimism – that we have thought through the situation before us and can justify our position.

Welcome to the world that I am describing as *furiously vegan*. I am in charge within this space, the master of my fate and captain of my soul. The spectrum of chronic and acute diseases plaguing too many of my fellow citizens cannot penetrate my natural health immunity. I AM too strong, fast, energetic, nourished, and mentally reinforced to be used and abused by the vulture-like corporations that are sucking the very life blood from individuals, families, communities, and the nation due to their parasitic medicine and healthcare practices.

I AM furiously vegan, and I thrive on Nature's perfect medicine. My medicine is the most delicious of all because I invested the time and effort to master the culinary arts. This exciting, fulfilling, and masterful life is the product of my *Kujichagulia* (self-determination) practices. My world is overflowing with an abundance, and I've surrounded myself with the most talented people of a generation. Yet, all that I experience is going according to an ever-expanding Master Plan. Thus, I shout to the four corners of the universe: *I AM FURIOUSLY VEGAN!*

That book of powerfully effective health and nutrition strategies has been out for about four plus one seasons. I cannot overstate just how correct were the instructions that have led me to the healthiest year I've enjoyed over the last decade. I would wish this feeling, this confidence, for every one of my family and community. I am not just aging gracefully. I am *reversing* the hallmarks of advanced age – noticeably returning all of my body markers to even before age 40. I keep my weight as close as possible to what I weighed at the peak of my adulthood, weighing in at 145 pounds (65.77 kg) at the age of 25 years.

Most adults in the USA gain and retain one pound yearly from that young age. Thus, today, 42 years after that age, it might be expected that my weight would be 187. My height of 5 feet and 8.5 inches would make me significantly overweight. Unfortunately, this is the case for too many men and women who graduated high school in 1973. In the years that have passed, being overweight and obese has become an epidemic within this society, and I have seen way too many of my age peers succumb to this deadly, energy-sapping trend.

Forty years ago, I committed to going in a different direction by giving up eating the Standard American Diet and even modified versions of it. I first went vegetarian in the early 1980s and intensified my focus to vegan by 1990. I'll never regret that decision and the demonstration of willpower that it took to remain strict over the decades that have followed.

FURIOUSLY VEGAN is my manifesto to celebrate and continuously rededicate my mind, body, and soul to this ultimate nutrition commitment. It has significantly changed my mental, physical, and spiritual fortitude.   The changes are profound:

- **FV** cemented my youthful senior status, and I am now living the superlative regarding my youthful high performance;

- It has proven the truth of the idea that "Old habits die hard, but new habits form quickly" – I am constantly reaffirming the practicality of new habit formation;

- No compromises mean no setbacks and no worries about seasonal acute inflammatory disorders that seem to plague so many people throughout the years;

- Keeping to a rigid schedule of detoxification with each changing season has done much to keep me in top form;

- *The Seven Principles of Optimal Health* are now rules for life;

- The right strategic supplementation regimen can make one feel and perform like a super man;

- I am currently living proof that we can revitalize our body systems on the cellular level, taking control over DNA expression and stem cell rejuvenation;

- It is not necessarily a given fact that men will lose their male potency with advancing age if they have a proper strategy for preserving youthful vitality.

- And that eating an exceptionally healthy nutritional cuisine never has to be dull, tasteless, boring, or too tedious to retain.

I love to eat and have a good time preparing the foods that tantalize and satisfy the need for tasty satiation. Becoming a primarily raw and live-food vegan that grows a substantial part of my weekly food intake was one of the greatest decisions for Life that I have committed to. Because of my success in this direction, so many other aspects of living have opened up to me. These include healthy longevity, immense creativity, a fully-functioning cognitive system, and avoiding forking over my hard-earned *labor-exchanged-dollars* (LEDs) to a medical-pharmaceutical healthcare establishment that wishes to profit from killing me slowly with their toxic chemotherapies. Nah... I ain't going out like that!

Living Superfood Longevity

Among the many keys to Life I have accumulated over the years is the value of mottos and affirmations. Another of my favorites is admonishing people to "Live long, love strong, and prosper."

Beyond merely kind words, these motifs inform, inspire and excite us to look for practical actions that consolidate these goals.

I now refer to a book I published in 2016 after three years of deep research and careful writing, ***LIVING SUPERFOOD LONGEVITY: Master the Possibilities of High-Quality Life Extension***. I often refer to this book as "an owner's manual for the adult body." One wouldn't think of owning a new automobile, computer, or other expensive mechanical technology without a good set of instructions to manage its function, maintenance, repair, and idiosyncrasies. Yet, most of the population doesn't follow the same mandate when fully comprehending how their body works and should be kept at optimal function.

Nature has a broad set of hard rules for longevity that are consistent, even across various species classes. In ***LONGEVITY***, I identified many of these rules and validated my hypothesis across numerous species of animals, reptiles, primates, and birds of similar species or stature. It has *always* proved consistent that **vegetarian animals outlived their omnivorous or carnivorous counterparts** by significant percentages.

We seek consistent rules, precise science, and natural biological precedents that serve our innate desires for longevity, disease resistance, and high physical performance as the foundation fo our health. Analogous to a luxury automobile, we seek longevity, reliability, and high performance from our human machine.

It is simply a matter of being aware of the functioning of the seventeen biological systems of the body and following Nature's rules for keeping things in proper functioning order. Once we have acquired this information and assembled it within our conscious understanding and organization, we can establish patterns of living and habits that secure our bio-integrity. A healthy future is ours to create masterfully.

Transforming Soul Food: For the Body, Mind, and Spirit

Culture is the ultimate determinant of behavior for the individual and the group, as it also transcends generations. Culture is the foundation of all great nations, empires, and civilizations throughout history. Culture is the encapsulation of any identifiable ethnic group's existence. To borrow from the lyrical expressions of Curtis Mayfield, culture is all-encompassing in one's life:

> *I'm your mama*
> *I'm your daddy, I'm that n***a*
> *In the alley, I'm your doctor*
> *When in need, want some coke?*
> *Have some weed, you know me*
> *I'm your friend—your main boy*
> *Thick and thin, I'm your pusherman*

Culture is the filler to all aspects of our individual and collective lives. This is true whether the culture is widespread or a tiny *subculture* within one or more larger cultures. Such is the stuff of the grand sciences of sociology, anthropology, history, and the evolution of civilizations. It cannot be overstated:

CULTURE IS!

Culture is composed of the following **Six Axioms**:

1. Language (including a person's name)
2. Spiritual expression/religion
3. Traditions (What did YOU do on the 4th of July?"
4. Historical perspective (a shared history, two opposite views)
5. Morals and values
6. Logical thinking and reasoning

Food is an essential component of cultural traditions. This is apparent and consistent around the world. Many cultures across the globe are celebrated for their unique culinary practices. Among favorite foods are Chinese, Indian, Thai, Ethiopian (my favorite), African, Cuban, Mexican, Italian, French, Jamaican, Persian, and Brazilian. One could even claim that American foods such as hamburgers, hot dogs, sugary beverages, and junk food are a distinct food culture – although one is aware that this uniquely American eating style is excessively toxic.

Among a subset of American foods is that distinction of her sable-skinned members. "Soul Food" is distinct to Negro heritage, although it is largely shared by poverty-class white people in the South and beyond. Soul Food has stood as the epitome of what I refer to as *chewicide*. In the book **Transforming Soul Food for the Body, Mind, and Spirit**, I share the following:

> Chewicide – When you absolutely positively know that you shouldn't be eating that stuff that you are eating, but you are hooked on the taste and thus justify continuing to do what you are accustomed to doing: That's Chewicide.

When your preferred nutritional lifestyle is directly associated with an increased risk of life-threatening chronic diseases like cancer, heart disease, clogged arteries, diabetes, high blood pressure, kidney failure, obesity, and mental illness: That's Chewicide.

When food is so absolutely, deliciously decadent that it literally is "to DIE for!" That's Chewicide.

Chewicide is a raging epidemic within the United States, and the standard African American diet, so-called SOUL FOOD, is the epitome of killer cuisine.[9]

We have all been taught that what you routinely eat can cause or prevent diseases and disorders. Once you have decided on the preferred outcome, finding the right pathway there should come naturally. The correctness of such a choice, combined with the power of the Will and the momentum of habit formation, can lead us to become masters of our dietary fate.

With this profound understanding, each meal becomes a divine healing session or another exhausting "dance with the devil." We know this now. Can we do better for our wise comprehension?

The Power of Habit

One of my favorite sayings is, **"Old habits die hard, but new habits form quickly."** I would be honored if you quoted me with that. With this in mind, I strongly advocate for everyone, especially our Big Up Manhood, to develop a powerful daily

---

[9] From the documentary CHEWICIDE, THE MOVIE, written and produced by Keidi Obi Awadu, 2014, Black Star Media Global

routine habit that complements your body, mind, spirit, and *massive transformative mission* (MTP).

Here is how I start each day:

- I wake with the sunrise, allowing the sun to fill the room;

- Upon rising, I turn on the morning news broadcast, drain my bladder and then begin 25 minutes of exercise with 150 reps each of knees to the chest, straight leg lifts, and sit-ups, separated by reverse planks;

- Make up my bed and organize my bedroom (eliminating chaos in my sleeping environment);

- My first bowel movement of the day is also my first daily reading experience; because I eat a lot of fiber, I speed read;

- I get on the scale and track my day-to-day weight carefully;

- During warmer weather, I will go out for 20 minutes of *high-impact interval training* (HIIT) for cardiovascular toning;

- Move into the office, start two computers, and launch the webcast program with recorded archives;

- Fix my morning hydration consisting of 1) 12 ounces of water with the juice of one-half fresh lemon, 1 ½ Tbl of raw, unfiltered cider vinegar, and 2 Tbl of goji berry juice, and 2) my morning tea, which includes green tea, black tea, cayenne pepper, ginger powder, cinnamon, turmeric, coconut oil, wild honey, and peppermint essential oil;

- I have some 44 anti-aging supplements in my extended arsenal, and most days, I will rotate about 9 to 12 of them into my daily routine; these I take along with the cider-lemon drink;

- For the next four hours, it is office time. This day is off to a magnificent start.

During the early afternoon hours, when the sunlight warms up a particular, habitual spot in my bedroom, I will engage in about three minutes of very deep breathing and then launch into my first set of push-ups for the day. I started engaging with intensive push-ups about a decade ago, achieving a remarkable "60 push-ups on my 60th birthday." I am very proud that just this week, I set a new lifetime record of 310 in a single set without pause. Some people refuse to believe that a man 67 years, five months, and eight days of age could do this. However, a number of my close associates have witnessed my push-ups.

I encourage everyone to adopt a challenging daily fitness routine. You will know in short order the many benefits of such daily disciplines. Every aspect of your vitality will be enhanced with such exercises.

The Disappearing Male in Modern Society

"Until they are confronted by the Lion, all hyenas believe they are the Alpha males." – Keidi Obi Awadu

The Explosive Documentary Film

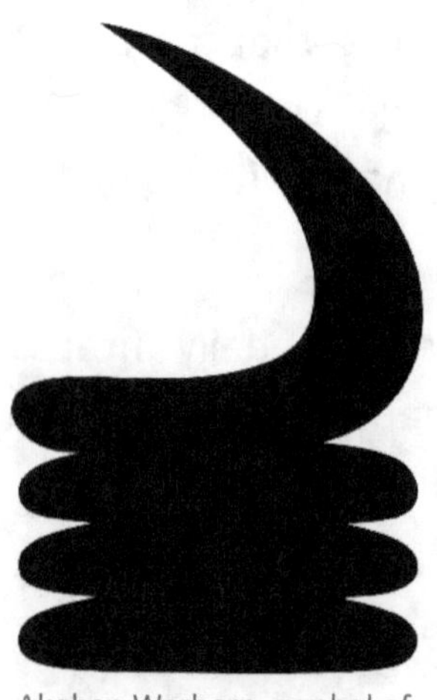

Akoben Warhorn, symbol of readiness, a call to action.

A 2008 Canadian documentary film written and directed by Marc De Guerre and produced by Alan Mendelsohn, *The Disappearing Male*, caused widespread alarm across the science community, environmental movement, health, and societal analysts. The film caught my attention early and prompted a heightened level of research regarding the shocking revelations about the decline of fertility impacting most men in modern societies.

Considered one of the top documentary films of the decade, here is a synopsis of the film:

The Disappearing Male is about one of the most important, and least publicized, issues facing the human species: the toxic threat to the male reproductive system.

The last few decades have seen steady and dramatic increases in the incidence of boys and young men suffering from genital deformities, low sperm count, sperm abnormalities and testicular cancer.

At the same time, boys are now far more at risk of suffering from ADHD, autism, Tourette's syndrome, cerebral palsy, and dyslexia.

The Disappearing Male takes a close and disturbing look at what many doctors and researchers now suspect are responsible for many of these problems: a class of common chemicals that are ubiquitous in our world.

Found in everything from shampoo, sunglasses, meat and dairy products, carpets, cosmetics and baby bottles, they are called "hormone mimicking" or "endocrine disrupting" chemicals and they may be starting to damage the most basic building blocks of human development.[10]

The film refers to the widespread introduction of endocrine-disrupting chemicals (EDCs), which we mentioned earlier in this book. The medical and pharmaceutical industries introduced some of these corrupters as they sought to create estrogen-mimicking drugs to affect pregnancy, chemotherapies, and other hormonal interventions.

Boys Will Be Girls Will Be Boys Will Be ???

This brings us to the notorious introduction in the 1940s of *diethylstilbesterol*. From the 1950s, it was widely proscribed to pregnant women to relieve pregnancy symptoms. It was discontinued because it caused havoc on the unborn fetuses exposed to the synthetic estrogen hormone.

---

[10] The Disappearing Male, a 2008 Canadian documentary film, written and directed by Marc De Guerre and produced by Alan Mendelsohn

Diethylstilbestrol (DES) is a synthetic form of the female hormone estrogen. It was prescribed to pregnant women between 1940 and 1971 to prevent miscarriage, premature labor, and related complications of pregnancy. The use of DES declined after studies in the 1950s showed that it was not effective in preventing these problems, although it continued to be used to stop lactation, for emergency contraception, and to treat menopausal symptoms in women.

In 1971, researchers linked prenatal (while in the womb, or in utero) DES exposure to a type of cancer of the cervix and vagina called clear cell adenocarcinoma in a small group of women. Soon after, the Food and Drug Administration (FDA) notified health care providers throughout the country that DES should not be prescribed to pregnant women. The drug continued to be prescribed to pregnant women in Europe until 1978.

DES is now known to be an endocrine-disrupting chemical, one of a number of substances that interfere with the endocrine system to potentially cause cancer, birth defects, and other developmental abnormalities.[11]

As we can determine from these revelations about the impact of DES and a vast spectrum of thousands of chemicals now known to be endocrine disrupters, there is a great reason to be alarmed about these developments on our bio-integrity and reproductive health. The terrible truth is that the corporate-dominated media, with its strong pro-pharma bias, has failed to properly inform the public and the problems with these drugs,

---

[11] Diethylstilbestrol (DES) Exposure and Cancer, What is DES?, National Cancer Institute

chemicals, and the spectrum of commonly-used products that negatively impact reproductive integrity. Likewise, government regulation has dismally failed to raise the alarm and inform the public regarding the real risks that continued introduction and usage of these chemicals pose to humanity.

I have examined the impact of estrogen-mimicking chemicals on the environment for many years. My 1997 book *MISSING ASSETS: Cultural, Biological, and Psychological Origins of Infertility* highlighted much about the manners by which these chemicals became ubiquitous and various mechanisms by which they were shown to undermine reproductive health.

Many scientific studies are pointing at a broad class of chemicals that have demonstrated the ability to interfere with the body's natural hormone (endocrine) system. These suspect chemicals, often referred to as *xenoestrogens* or *endocrine-disrupting chemicals* (EDCs), have been linked to many of the same discomforts of chemical birth control and demonstrate carcinogenic (cancer-causing) abilities and lead to infertility. EDCs have become so widespread within industrialized societies that a terrible plague of compromised fertility has become evident — affecting not only humans but animals alike.

I first explored these issues in a series of articles compiled into the **Conscious Rasta Report** entitled *POPULATION WAR: REPORT FROM THE FRONTLINE.* Additionally, other substances which have demonstrated this endocrine-disrupting capability include the artificial hair known as Kanekalon™, lipstick and other cosmetics, herbicides, fungicides, paint, spermicides, food additives, artificial hormones and steroids, synthetic birth control, organochlorines, liquid detergents, plastic food packaging, and synthetic fabrics. Within the environment of highly industrialized nations, these chemicals are increasingly pervasive. Because scientists have raised these alarms for several decades, business and political leadership are apparently sacrificing the long-term reproductive health of humans and animal species for short-term profits and convenience. What a foolish endeavor![12]

We have learned much more about how these chemicals have permeated the food chain, including meat, poultry, eggs, dairy, and many processed foods. Yet, even more tragically, the number of known endocrine-disrupting chemicals commonly used in modern society continues to increase.

As information (and misinformation) proliferates in the media about endocrine-disrupting chemicals (EDCs), so do questions about where they are found and how we might be exposed to them through eating, drinking, breathing, or touching.

Answers to these questions are not always simple. There are nearly 85,000 man-made chemicals in the world, many of which people come into contact with every day. Only about one percent of them have been studied for safety; however, 1,000 or more of these chemicals may

---

[12] MISSING ASSETS: Cultural, Biological, and Psychological Origins of Infertility, by Keidi Awadu, 1997, pgs.48-50

be EDCs based on their probable endocrine-interfering properties.[13]

This excerpt just shared is from *The Endocrine Society*. The extensive report lists a few of the thousands of chemicals that disrupt hormonal functioning in humans and other species. These include (but are not limited to):

- **Brominated flame retardants** (BFRs) are used in electronics, clothing, and furniture such as sofas and mattresses;

- **Polychlorinated biphenyls** (PCBs) are used in thousands of industrial and commercial applications due to their flame resistance, insulating properties, and chemical stability.

- **Phthalates** interfere with androgen production (testosterone), a hormone critical in male development and relevant to females. Phthalates are present in hundreds of products, including food and beverage containers and plastic wraps. People are exposed to these EDCs when they leach into foods or are released when containers are microwaved.

- **Bisphenol A** (BPA) is among the best-known and most pervasive EDCs. In humans, it is linked to reduced egg quality and lack of viability among women seeking fertility treatment.

- **Children's Products** – EDCs are being gradually regulated or banned in children's toys, games, and accessories such as baby bottles. However, older products manufactured outside of the United States and European Union or battery-operated may be of particular concern.

---

[13] Common EDCs and Where They Are Found, The Endocrine Society,

- **Pesticides and Herbicides** – Many pesticides are designed to be toxic to pests' nervous or reproductive systems and act by disrupting endocrine systems. Such chemicals are also EDCs because insect and animal endocrine systems are similar.

- **EDCs Contaminating Our Water and Food Supply** – Per- and polyfluoroalkyl substances (PFAS) are artificial chemicals used as oil and water repellents and coatings for common products, including cookware, carpets, and textiles.

I trust that you now have a much larger perspective about the role of these endocrine disruptors in contributing to the continued compromise of the definitions of male and man, female and woman. As a member of the Baby Boom generation, I have been a direct observer of these corrupting changes in society and health over my nearly-completed seven decades of life. I am not the only one to be extremely alarmed about these affairs.

It was Rachael Carson's 1962 book **SILENT SPRING** that is considered to be a hallmark of the modern environmental movement. In the book, she exposed the mutations in animal species' reproductive integrity that signaled an alarm that these same chemicals would increasingly undermine human fertility. Nations should have heeded Rachael Carson's warnings:

Silent Spring, is a nonfiction book written by Rachel Carson that became one of the most-influential books in the modern environmental movement. Published in 1962, Silent Spring was widely read by the general public and became a New York Times best seller. The book provided the impetus for tighter control of pesticides and has been honored on many lists of influential books...

Documenting the many harmful effects pesticides have on the environment, Carson argued that pesticides should properly be called "biocides" because of their impact on organisms other than the target pests. Specifically, she noted the harm DDT inflicted on bird populations and warned of a future spring characterized by the lack of birdsong. She highlighted the fact that DDT was classified as a chemical carcinogen implicated in causing liver tumors in mice and accused representatives of the chemical industry of spreading disinformation contradicted by scientific research. She also accused government officials of uncritically accepting the chemical industry's claims of safety and, more radically, questioned the then-dominant paradigm of scientific progress and the philosophical belief that man was destined to exert control over nature.[14]

I will frequently point to the undermining role that media and government regulators serve to cover up the havoc with reproductive health posed by the contamination from these chemicals. Additionally, the role of mass media and entertainment in swapping out masculine and feminine role models and characters in their entertainment fare cannot be ignored. I am probably not the only one disturbed by the encroachment of masculinized females into traditional roles that we've grown accustomed to in cinema, television, and other entertainment. You may have even heard of proposals to portray the *consummate machismo character of James Bond* into a female actor – it's already been going on for years as

---

[14] Silent Spring work by Carson, Written by Sarah E. Boslaugh, Encyclopedia Britannica, Last Updated: Jan 24, 2023

women come to assume more super masculine agents of state security in these fictional worlds.

This represents a century-old comprehensive eugenics scheme to destroy families and the resultant fertility of targeted groups. We witness a widespread social engineering scheme to change the very nature of societies to reduce the world's growing population. I hope you can see this in a greater context upon reading this chapter and this book.

Radical Feminism Assaults the World

Given the number of ways that aggressive feminists are assaulting our autonomy, it should be easer for black leaders to gain a functional perspective of the undermining impact that western feminist imperialism has had on our people. A cunning, clandestine conspiracy seems to be in place to displace all aspects of Black Manhood and to substitute in its place a new feminist hierarchy. This assault has been going on against western culture for a century and more. Where it began as an expression of women's desire for an equality of human, economic, political, and social opportunities, it has now mutated to a more sinister scheme do dominate all aspects of these societal functions.

There exist certain bizarre alliances to collaborate with the feminist radicals, that receive disproportionate advocacy from black politicians, media pundits, and other higher-profile Afri-Amer leaders. Two of these, which run directly contradictory to the group's survival self-interests, are *championing abortion* and promoting the legitimacy of *gender-nonconformity*.

In these liberal democracies, people have been extended the choice to cancel their future. In such a society, people have the right to attempt sexual rituals within an expanding variety of unnatural configurations. Toward the aim of preserving the group for generations of survival, these two behaviors are contradictory, as are other anti-fertility lifestyle patterns.

Much of this procreative degeneration is the result of radical feminism disseminated from a people whose fertility has crashed – they want to take as many of out with them as will concede.

The Eugencists' Agenda

Lest we should not have a long-term perspective on what is happening, we have had more than a century of strategies and tactics to limit childbirths among the so-called *undesirable population* within white-dominated societies. We recall these shocking pronouncements from the 1944 book by the Nobel Prize-winning Swedish economist Gunnar Myrdal, himself an acknowledged eugenicist, revealed in the largest study of Blacks in America ever published:

"If we forget about the means, for the moment, and consider only the quantitative goal for Negro population policy, there is no doubt that the *overwhelming majority of white Americans desire that there be as few Negroes as possible in America*. If the Negroes could be eliminated from America or greatly decreased in numbers, this would meet the whites' approval— *provided that it could be accomplished by means which are also approved*. Correspondingly, an increase of the proportion of Negroes in the American population is commonly looked upon as undesirable... Commonly it is considered a great misfortune for America that Negro slaves were ever imported. The presence of Negroes in

> America today is usually considered as a "plight" of the nation... [15]

Indeed, Myrdal's book, which the Carnegie Foundation commissioned during World War II, was delivered to the office of the President as part of the nation's national security concerns that Blacks would align with the nation's foreign enemies to serve as a "Fifth Column" to attack the country from within. In this excerpt, what is proposed fits the legal definition of genocide.

Three pages later, in the same chapter, **Negro Population**, various strategies for carrying out the elimination of all or the majority of the African-descended population in the U.S., the following revealed the *means* by which genocide might occur:

> In our further discussion of the means in Negro population policy we might start out from the desire of the politically dominant white population to get rid of the Negroes. This is a goal difficult to reach by approved means, and the desire has never been translated into action directly, and probably never will be. All the most obvious means go strongly against the American creed. The Negroes cannot be killed off. Compulsory deportation would infringe upon personal liberty in such a radical fashion that it is excluded. Voluntary exportation of Negroes could not be carried on extensively because of unwillingness on the part of recipient nations as well as on the part of the American Negroes themselves, who usually do not want to leave the country but prefer to stay and fight it out here.

---

[15] AN AMERICAN DILEMMA: The Negro Problem and Modern Democracy, by Gunnar Myrdal, Harper & Brothers, 1944. Pg. 167

Neither is it possible to effectuate the goal by keeping up the Negro death rate.   A high death rate is an unhumanitarian and undemocratic way to restrict the Negro population and, in addition, expensive to society and dangerous to the white population.   The only possible way of decreasing Negro population is by means of controlling fertility...

In the final analysis *all these theoretically possible policies to effectuate the white desire to decrease the Negro population are blocked by the American Creed* (except birth control which, however, is largely attached to other ends).[16] [Myrdal, 1944 pg. 170]

How long has this "American Creed" affected the lives of U.S. Blacks? In 1852 Frederick Douglass called it "hollow mockery."

Over the thirty years I have been writing about demographics, population control, and related topics, my archive of such damning indictments of eugenicists has amassed quite an arsenal of their worst ideologies. The following insights from a journalist comrade exposing these satanic intentions are critical to our understanding:

[In order] "for population control to succeed, a great deal more must be done than to merely establish family planning centers and to provide surreptitious funding for local advocacy campaigns.   An entire spectrum of variables affecting the desire to have children must be influenced – from basic economics and government programs to family relations, personal expectations,

---

[16] ANALYSIS OF MYRDAL'S "AN AMERICAN DILEMMA" excerpted from HIGH CRIMES OF MURDER, by Keidi Obi Awadu, 1999, pg. 17

lifestyle, cultural tradition, concepts of land sharing and private ownership, wealth production systems, ethical standards, and even religious beliefs. Taboos must be breached, the bonds that unite family and community must be undermined, and sufficient disruption must occur to literally disorient the targeted communities and make them vulnerable to the imposition of external cultural forces.[17]

Social engineering is a method by which powerful entities seek to control and dominate large segments of people and implement strategies to impact the lives of large parts of the population. They aim to create certain predetermined and desired outcomes that benefit themselves as the engineers and undermine the masses' sovereignty, independence, and unrestricted development.

The rich always seem to want more. Despite great wealth across the nation, it is increasingly concentrated in the coffers of an insatiable wealthy class. The scoundrels of the late 19th and early 20th Centuries have returned with a vengeance. <u>Welcome to the New Age of the Robber Barons</u>. Their lust for wealth and power seems to be insatiable. Unfortunately, efforts on the part of the shrinking middle class seem too often to only focus on making their way into the *uber-rich* rather than finding ways to spread the wealth of the nation to the widest possible numbers so that we all can afford the basic necessities of comfort, security, health and nutrition, and other amenities a wealthy nation provides.

---

[17] PROPAGANDA, CULTURAL IMPERIALISM & POPULATION CONTROL: Ideological Communications in the Southern Hemisphere, from the Information Project For Africa

The World Is Mine

What is needed is a prescription of how to deal with this ideology of unchecked greed, genocidal manipulation, the constant trampling of our civic and human rights, and the grand theft of the wealth produced from our labors. We need a manifesto to serve as our protocol for countering doctrines and stimulate each of us, along with our masses, to resist. From my 1999 book, ***THE ROAD TO POWER: Seven Steps to an African Global Order***, comes the following inspiring manifesto for sovereign, self-determined development:

We acknowledge and appreciate the positive contributions of different civilizations to the progress of humanity. We also rebuke our society's activities and others' that have caused destruction or hindered humanity's progress. We will form alliances with other cultural groups only when interests are complementary.

Though we are followers of the "**Race First**" philosophy of Marcus Garvey, we recognize that we would always show respect to those other ethnic groups that show respect to us, as did the Honorable Marcus Garvey.

We do not dislike others simply for who they are, but we do not tolerate our community's disrespect and injury. We stand against ignorance, yet we are intolerant of those whose actions are injurious to our enlightened self-interests. Toward this end, we will actively defend our family against insults and injuries from hostile external groups, and we will refrain from insulting and injuring those groups outside of our own, which have not expressed such aggression against us.

But for those whose intentions would come into antagonistic contradiction with our visions of empowerment and enlightenment, we vow to fight actively and with all malice to defeat those intentions and, if necessary, to eliminate any groups who consistently express hostile intent.

Toward this end, we vow not to be bombastic without action, not to be hypocritical, and not to be weak or cowardly. Thus, in defense of Life, we are willing to commit our lives and, if necessary, to take lives as required to preserve Life within our African village.

Gender Confusion & Bio-Logical War

"Teaching children to deny biology is maddening. Telling them they get to choose if you're a girl or boy, or both or neither, because they may have been incorrectly assigned an identity at birth, that's a man made idea,"
— Dr. Miriam Grossman[18]

Population Wars / Culture Wars

Over three decades, one of the most frequent themes I have written about is demographics. Shifting population numbers matter, and this topic can be approached from many different angles. Due in large part to my biosciences background, combined with a decade of association with the Washington, DC think tank *The Information Project For Africa* (IPFA), I have long found the study of people numbers, how they impact the fate of nations, and their convergence with reproductive biological integrity.

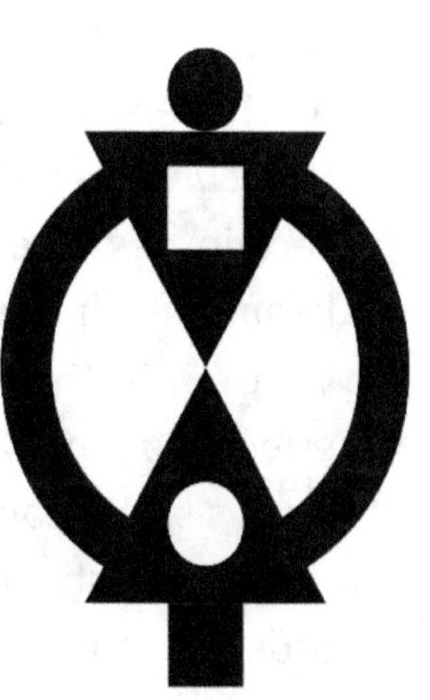

Boa me na mmoa:
Take into consideration the conspiracy about a person.

The following are some of these insights as they have appeared in my books since the late 1980s.

- **Rule # 1: SURVIVAL OF THE FITTEST** — and key to the survival of any people, be they an ethnic group, nation, or race, is continued procreation. Our beloved creator blesses

---

[18] Experts: We must defeat gender ideology and protect children, AMERICAN NEWS: Post Millennial, Sept. 12, 2022

nations with fruitful generations or barrenness if the people have fallen out of favor with God. But, even for those who do produce significant numbers of childbirths, if the structure of the community is weak or disorientated, if parenting skills are sufficiently lacking or underdeveloped, or if the genetic material which has coalesced in the child is weak or defective — the end result is a failure of the necessary natural procreation process. That is a violation of Rule # 1: Survival of the fittest.[19]

- In a groundbreaking 1993 work entitled **The Trojan Horse Analysis**, I demonstrated how the most popular rap and hip-hop videos were encoded with what I termed the *"Twelve Reoccurring Negative Themes."* Constant repetition of certain negative themes within the videos was subliminally beaming self-destructive ideas into the minds of vulnerable youth. Further analysis following the rules of cause and effect has proven the correctness of the Trojan Horse Analysis. We can now witness evidence of a terrifying set of negative behaviors absolutely contrary to the nature of urban youth or the community from which they sprang.

- These 12 themes which I articulated included techniques that came straight out of the U.S. Army's psychological warfare catalog, such as subliminal programming methods aimed at demonization and criminalization of the enemy (urban youth), hypnotic techniques to create chaos, and a centrally-coordinated anti-youth propaganda campaign throughout the mainstream press. Before the Trojan Horse Analysis, I was unaware anyone had taken on a scientific and

---

[19] RAP, HIP-HOP, AND THE NEW WORLD ORDER: Planned Chaos in Youth Music Culture, by Keidi Obi Awadu, 1996

psychological analysis of the widely promoted rap and hip-hop videos to defend the community. Too many criticized the youth music culture, blaming the hip-hop generation for things beyond the youth's ability to instigate themselves. No, there were bigger forces at work here, and they were largely escaping criticism from those silly politicians, ministers, and other critics who were making all the noise. Breaking down this social disruption occurring within the hip-hop generation in a scientific approach and understanding it as such, this mayhem becomes quite alarming, and the consequences of this make it intolerable.[20]

- Because white women worldwide have produced the most dramatic plunge in childbirths than has ever been witnessed, Western security agencies are committed to policies intended to address a predicted loss of political, economic, and military influence. The significance of this set of consequences must not be under-appreciated.

- To discount this reproductive predicament for worldwide European culture is not to be able to become aware of the factors which tie so many seemingly-random and chaotic activities together. To misunderstand the population imperative is to exist within the illusion that mere hard work and honesty will provide a good life for most of the world's population. But when it comes down to managing the world's population from its present level of 5.8 billion persons down to a preferred target of as few as 2-4 billion, and such targeting is well documented, this is not going to be a pretty scenario. Such a radical population control program would require the deaths of young and old. The

---

[20] Ibid., pg. 3

ideal target would be young women entering their prime procreative years. This would also include baby girls and boys. Yes, the face of population control is discriminating and ugly.[21]

- One finds it shocking to recognize the myriad of ways by which modern man and woman have deviated from nature and found themselves on the short end of procreation. Moreover, the introduction into developed societies of social trends such as homosexuality, widespread infertility, synthetic birth control, less rigid family structures, environmentalism, cybersex, male-female conflict, and increasingly delayed first childbirth has negatively impacted or will shortly, fertility in these nations.[22]

- Having read this report [Population War], you have been forewarned. Thus to continue with business-as-usual is to invite "race suicide" and the disappearance of your own culture. Don't procrastinate on this issue. Study these issues further and make an effort to teach those around you. Build progressive action agenda based on firm research.[23]

- While we all need to recognize the importance of individual will, there is a collective will that has traditionally been of greater significance. In Africa, and other traditional societies, this has always been known as the concept of "The Village." The Village stands as a broader family or clan entity. Within such a society, certain individual functions were relegated to the needs of the collective.

---

[21] Ibid, pg. 11
[22] POPULATION WAR: Report from the Frontline, by Keidi Obi Awadu, 1996
[23] Ibid, pg. 62

- Within the Village, each child born was looked upon as a source of wealth to the clan, and women who birthed the greatest number of healthy children were elevated to a higher status within the group.

- Within the Village, a male was brought to manhood through a complicated ritual process of education, instruction from older men, and initiation. Only after initiation could he engage in sexual activity with a childbearing-age female.

- "[F]or population control to succeed, a great deal more must be done than to merely establish family planning centers and to provide surreptitious [covert] funding for local advocacy campaigns. An entire spectrum of variables affecting the desire to have children must be influenced – from basic economics and government programs to family relations, personal expectations, lifestyle, cultural tradition, concepts of land sharing and private ownership, wealth production systems, ethical standards, and even religious beliefs. Taboos must be breached, the bonds that unite family and community must be undermined, and sufficient disruption must occur to literally disorient the targeted communities and make them vulnerable to the imposition of external cultural forces.[24]

- "Family planning [population control] seeks to influence human behavior. Motivation is therefore an important part of any approach to the population problem. This requires

---

[24] MISSING ASSETS: Cultural, Biological, and Psychological Origins of Infertility, by Keidi Obi Awadu, 1997, citing the document PROPAGANDA, CULTURAL IMPERIALISM & POPULATION CONTROL: Ideological Communications in the Southern Hemisphere, from the Information Project For Africa

understanding of cultural, social, psychological and economic forces..."[25]

- As stated earlier, it is sometimes hard to distinguish the activities of hostile external groups against a targeted enemy from behaviors adopted by the subjected group that contribute to the weakening or demise of the group. I have written about such unconsciously adopted self-limiting behaviors in several books focusing on behavior modification and social engineering. The techniques and methodologies of those instigating these campaigns comprise what I have long referred to as "population wars/culture wars." Under this state of organized affairs, members of the target society adopt patterns of behaviors, actions, logic, and morality, undermining their ability to survive and thrive within the nation. These targeted communities take on such behaviors both consciously and unconsciously.[26]

Across the nearly four dozen books I have written, themes related to demographics, population control, cultural manipulation, childbearing age youth, civilization clashes, scientific futurism, and fertility shifts have been dominating themes, upon which we all must continue to learn.

From Eugenics to Gender Neutralization

Over the past decade, within the U.S. and other western culture-impacted societies, subjects relative to the blending of gender identity have become mainstream. Two of the

---

[25] POLICY DETERMINATION: POPULATION AND FAMILY PLANNING PROGRAMS, which appeared as part of a larger Government Accounting Office (GAO) report, November 1967, cited in MISSING ASSETS, 1997

[26] FADE TO BLACK: The Passing of a Great Race, by Keidi Obi Awadu 2020, pg 15

terminologies introduced within these ideologies are **gender identity disorder** and **gender dysphoria**.[27]

News media are increasingly musing about these radical shifts in society, as the following examples are illustrative:

> **Daniel Goleman**, *The New York Times* — "The main symptoms of gender identity disorder include not just a strong wish to be the opposite sex and unhappiness about one's actual sex, but also distress about this predicament that is so severe it interferes with the child's functioning."[28]

> **Louis J. Gooren,** *The New England Journal of Medicine* -- "Manifestations of gender identity disorder range from simply living as a member of the opposite sex to partial or maximal physical adaptation through hormonal and surgical treatment."[29]

The authoritative online dictionary Merriam-Webster defines *gender dysphoria* as "a distressed state arising from conflict between a person's gender identity and the sex the person has or was identified as having at birth."

We note that there has been a rising reluctance to accept this gender confusion outside of the political, psychological, and sociological advocacy spreading it across the national culture.

Gender Identity Disorder, defined as a disorder in 1978, has seized up pressures of modern *political correctness* to no longer

---

[27] Gender Identity Disorder / Gender Dysphoria, Merriam-Webster Dictionary, 3 Feb., 2023

[28] The 'Wrong' Sex: A New Definition Of Childhood Pain, by Daniel Goleman, NY Times, Mar. 1994

[29] Care of Transsexual Persons, by Louis J. Gooren, The New England Journal of Medicine, Mar. 2011

be seen as a maladaptive psychiatric condition. This phenomenon of normalizing what insurance companies regarded as a pre-existing pathological condition is a relatively recent social-political evolution, not biological.

I put forth that this change reflects a deliberate eugenicist scheme that also conforms to clandestine machinations of the population controllers that push their *satanic* anti-childbirth agenda.

When this same inquiry into "gender identity disorder" is put to the socially liberal *Wikipedia*, it appears as the following aberration, which includes dropping the notion that this behavior represents an *atypical psychological state*:

> Gender identity is the personal sense of one's own gender. Gender identity can correlate with a person's assigned sex or can differ from it. In most individuals, the various biological determinants of sex are congruent, and consistent with the individual's gender identity. Gender expression typically reflects a person's gender identity, but this is not always the case. While a person may express behaviors, attitudes, and appearances consistent with a particular gender role, such expression may not necessarily reflect their gender identity. The term gender identity was coined by psychiatry professor Robert J. Stoller in 1964 and popularized by psychologist John Money.[30]

This excerpt reflects the corruption of social, cultural, and wellness norms, which an increasing number of scholars have raised in castigating Wikipedia as a reliable and trustworthy

---

[30] Gender Identity, from Wikipedia, The Free Encyclopedia

reference source. I agree with these critics. I often refer to the online encyclopedia to determine the reverse perspective of what I believe to be true and correct. Therefore, because of social liberalism and other scientific and political biases, I caution that you use Wiki as a source at your own risk.

The Alphabet Agenda / Queer Empire

The following was recently sent to me from an associate that was attached to this disturbing note:

Here's a screenshot of one of the pages I am visiting that is asking for "gender" identification. You and I spoke about this last time we were online and you commented that you wanted to include in your next book. This is the first one I have encountered since we spoke.

Which of the following is your current gender identity? [31]

- o   Cisgender female (born female. identifies as female)
- o   Cisgender male (born male, identifies as male)
- o   Trans female/trans woman
- o   Trans male/trans man
- o   Genderqueer/gender non-conforming
- o   Prefer not to answer
- o   Prefer to self-identify (What gender do you identify with?)

Something has gone shockingly off track within this current generation. The have been numerous cautions and warnings about the pace of population increase on this planet since the 18th Century. I have written extensively over three decades

---

[31] Survey Request from the National Recruiting Center, Field Work, 2023

about these concerns in a half-dozen books; I do not wish to recap these hysterical pronouncements again in this book.

What we do know is that very powerful people from across the spectrum of societal governance, leadership, security establishments, and environmentalists have claimed that they cannot imagine the continued growth of economic viability if the global population crosses certain thresholds over the coming three decades.

I don't believe their hype and have been refuting it for a long time. My problem is that I do not wield the kind of authoritative influence that these wealthy schemers are able to muster. They have immense resources at the availability. The propaganda that they produce, distribute, and sustain has a powerful effect on the general mindset. They are quite determined to control global population at a time in history where the greatest demographic dividend is now passing firmly into the advantage of a global African population that was suppressed by external forces for the last 2600 years.

Intending on steering humanity off this course of the childbirth advantage moving firmly to the residents of the southern hemisphere, these population manipulators are trying every way imaginable to change the nature of culture that has prioritized children, family, expansive community, and every advantage that society would give to reproductive-age youth.

Their propaganda and mind controlling influence across media promote all manners of procreative collapse. They have normalized bizarre behaviors such as the legitimization of a mal seeking sexual fulfillment in another male's digestive tract. Females nesting with others of their own kind, and a broad class of confused people who are clueless as to how the processes of replication of the species is supposed to work and are thus experimenting with whatever pops into their mind.

Things have gone array. The fabled Humpty Dumpty has fallen from his natural reproductive grace for an increasing number of densely populated societies, while "all the King's horses and all the King's men" seem clueless how to make things right for their team. Therefore, if they can no longer enjoy the benefits of the fertility advantage, then they seem to want to deny it for everyone.

Many of us are repulsed at what we are witnessing with this rapid and widespread degeneration of natural reproductive biology, degeneration and decadence all around. As an Elder, considered wise and esteemed, I find it appalling, although I have had several decades to examine these trends and comprehend the forces behind it. We have some of the population controllers most revealing confessions and motivations in our possession and many of their ideas are shocking. Note the following from one of the top U.S. national security operatives of the 1960s and 1970s who worked in the Lyndon Johnson White House security circles and later for the World Bank, Robert McNamara, speaking in 1979:

"There are only two possible ways in which a world of 10 billion people can be averted. Either the current birth rates must come down more quickly. Or the current death rates must go up. There is no other way. There are, of course, many ways in which the death rates can go up. In a thermonuclear age, war can accomplish it very quickly and decisively. Famine and disease are nature's ancient checks on population growth, and neither one has disappeared from the scene. Indeed, they have been quite active in recent years. But modern medicine and agriculture have artificially and temporarily reduced the effective impact of these two natural phenomena. In the long run, however, population growth must be matched by resource growth, or we will find ourselves in a world of famine and disease.[32]

Forty years later the various mechanisms of population control are firmly in place. At this point it is somewhat comforting that many national populations are resisting this manipulation by the western security establishments and their many operatives across the collaborative spectrum. However, those of that oppose this sinister agenda cannot drop our guard. The plot to deny the African continent the chance to reap the rewards of the demographic dividend for the majority of the 21st Century and beyond is too well established and lavishly funded. We need to pay particular attention to their methodologies that utilize mass media, culture wars, and subliminal manipulation to trick us out of our empowering destiny.

When we examine the strategies of population control through social engineering, deft use of communications initiatives to accomplish their manipulation must be seriously considered:

Nothing can be left to chance. To be effective, an intervention in the media must be thorough, careful, persistent, and extravagant. It must be capable of penetrating the minds of the audience at the subconscious, as well as the conscious level. It must systematically create an illusion on a massive scale, while

---

[32] "Population Growth and World Food Supplies: Implications and Outlook. Robert S. McNamara, speech delivered at the annual meeting of the International Planned Parenthood Federation in Nairobi, Kenya, on November 8, 1979

at the same time remaining discreet enough to give the impression that the false doctrine represents a spontaneous change in the target society itself.[33]

Bringing this back to the topic of this chapter, the rapid diffusion of ideologies from aggressive western feminism have come to dominate the rapid expansion of what we call "the alphabet agenda" (LBGTQIA+, etc.). I have cited extensive data within this report and recent books on how the doctrine of anti-fertility is doubling in the American population every 20-year birth generation. Reportedly, the highest percentage of American ethnic subcategories that is buying into this degeneration is Gen-Y African American females.

In the 2020 book ***FADE TO BLACK: The Passing of a Great Race***, I warned that the data on shrinking demographics for Blacks in the U.S. had fallen significantly below replacement. I showed conclusively that the decline in fertility in our group between 1975 and 2020 if continued for the next 45 years on the same exponentially declining trajectory, would signal the real disappearance of our subgroup by the year 2065. The single issue of widespread abortion among our people would be the prime factor of such a dramatic demographic collapse.

Theoretically, it is not yet too late to reverse this trend. However, I don't think there is any possibility of recovery without significant input from the fertility abundance that is the current advantage to childbearing age populations across Sub-Saharan Africa. Whether we can call upon that opportunity is not a guarantee. Moreover, this redemption will require a major paradigm shift in the cultural alignment of Blacks in western societies.

---

[33] MIND CONTROL by Keidi Obi Awadu, Conscious Rasta Press, 1996, pg. 18

Abortion: Fifty Years of Race Suicide
On the Frontline Against Infanticide

From the early 1990s, I have consistently projected a hostile stance against the unholy practice of abortion. At the earliest declaration of this position, I was a very lonely voice within the Afri-Amer community. I was strongly influenced to such a vocal stance by my admission to the DC-based international think tank, the *Information Project For Africa*, which, sadly, no longer exists.

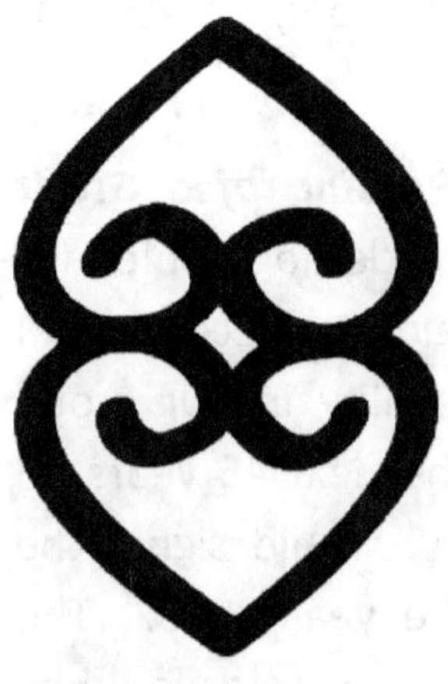

Asase Yaa symbolizes the Akan goddess of fertility, love, peace, and truth.

The I.P.F.A. was a collective of over 300 journalists from around the world that investigated issues of Pan-African sustainable development, demographics, population control, covert security affairs, and a broad manner of schemes designed to keep Africans and other darker peoples subservient spiritually culturally, politically, economically, socially, and judicially to the historically colonizing peoples.

I learned so much through collaboration with fellow journalists and researchers from the I.P.F.A. They found great value in one of my earliest books, ***ANOTHER LOADED NEEDLE: The SPF66 Malaria Vaccine and the Plot to Decimate the Population of Africa***. Through the Information Project For Africa, I became one of the first African-centered scholars in the U.S. to have a visible presence across the then-new platform of the Internet.

During this time of affiliation with IPFA, I was intensely tutored in the scholarship of population, fertility, the battle for child birthing, and the role of demographics in determining the rise and fall of civilization throughout history. One particular focus for which I was particularly equipped was the *future implications* of demographics in guiding the course of the planet for the next two centuries and more.

- "Abortion in America has contributed to the greatest decline in black population since the first black slaves arrived in the Americas in the 1600s. According to U.S. census data, there were 18,871,831 black American citizens in 1960. Since Roe v. Wade legalized abortion in 1973, abortion has killed an estimated 20 million black babies — more than the entire black population of 1960."[34]

- "Is Planned Parenthood purposely marketing abortion to minorities? According to author Willis Krumholz at The *Federalist*, Planned Parenthood's business model promotes that strategy because it's in their financial best interest to do so. Furthermore, he proposes that data showing the harm done to poor and minority women has been whitewashed by the formerly reliable Guttmacher Institute in order to protect the abortion giant."[35]

- "In the United States, black children are aborted at more than three times the rate of white children; Hispanic children are aborted at one and a half times the rate. Whatever the intentions of Planned Parenthood, abortion is eliminating an incommensurate number of minority children."[36]

---

[34] Abortion's twisted logic of racism during Black History Month, by Catherine Davis and Bradley Mattes, Washington Examiner, February 28, 2020
[35] More Evidence Planned Parenthood Markets Abortion to Minorities, by Susan W. Enouen, Life Issues Institute, June 2016
[36] Abortion and Race

- If you think abortion is a fundamental human right, perhaps you celebrate the fact that black children are being sacrificed to this privilege at quadruple the rate of whites. But if abortion is an act of violence that kills an innocent human being, then something far more sinister is at work here.[37]

- "[A]bortion ratios decreased among non-Hispanic white women but not among women in any other racial/ethnic group. For non-Hispanic white women, the abortion ratio decreased 3%, whereas the abortion ratio increased 4% for non-Hispanic black women..." [Abort73, Dec. 2012]

- Among white women, there were 138 abortions for every 1,000 births. Correspondingly, among black women, there were 501 abortions for every 1,000 births; this disparity representing a ratio of 3.63 abortions to African American women to every one for European American women. [2012]

- Though African-Americans represent 12% of the population, they represent 35% of aborted children [2012]

In my 2020 book **_FADE TO BLACK: The Passing of a Great Race_**, I tried to put into context that misaligned focus of our public on the attrition rate of killings by law enforcement, compared to far more deadly forces impacting Afri-Amers. In the chapter entitled **The Myth of Black Lives Matter**, I shared the following statistics:

Compared to nationally reported killings of our group's members by law enforcement actions, Blacks kill others of our group each year **at a ratio of 8.85-to-1**. Compared

---

For decades, abortion has disproportionately eliminated minority babies, from Abort73 online, July 09, 2020

[37] Seeing Abortion in Black and White, Abort73, December 2012

to law enforcement killings, **bad medical practices kill Blacks at a rate of 585-to-1**. **Abortion terminates black pregnancies at a rate of 1,067-to-1** annually within the United States.

The demonic duplicity that the liberals that support these industries of *infanticide* perpetuate directly in our face is appalling; made worse by the coopting of black feminists (including feminized males), complicit in this eugenics genocide. This gross hypocrisy was pointed out by the anti-abortion group *Abort73*, as many were commemorating **Black Out Tuesday** (#blackouttuesday) across Instagram and other social media:

More significantly, Planned Parenthood's corporate Twitter account issued the following statement on Monday:

"We're devastated, grieving, and outraged by violence against Black lives. We must continue to demand accountability, justice, and an end to the inequity that continues to define every moment of life for Black America from the racist institutions that uphold white supremacy."[38]

The author of this devastatingly revealing research posting, Michael Spielman, condemned the sinister hypocrisy of Planned Parenthood's corporate office on the event of Black Out Tuesday. I couldn't think of any better way to describe this sordid affair:

Whether you agree with that statement or not—which asserts that U.S. police departments are "racist

---

[38] PLANNED PARENTHOOD KILLS BLACK BABIES. LEGALLY. EN MASSE. By Michale Spielman, Abort73, June 3, 2020

institutions that uphold white supremacy," it's who's making the statement that makes it so damned duplicitous. Talk about the pot calling the kettle black! Last year, police officers in the United States killed nine unarmed black persons—and 19 unarmed white persons. By comparison, Planned Parenthood killed approximately 131,000 unarmed black babies (in 2018) and 121,000 unarmed white babies. Think about those numbers for a moment.

Think about these numbers for more than a moment. Consider this eugenicist plot in the context of a century and more of racist population control policies that reach across the entire spectrum of hostile western societies. Consider Planned Parenthood from the revelations that the founder of its precursor, Margaret Sanger was a noted eugenicists who initiated **The Negro Project**, to coopt black leadership in reducing our fertility, in the mid-1920s.

As revealed in *FADE TO BLACK*, at least 22.7 million abortions to black women between 1973 and 2020, has reduced the potential population of our U.S. group by 42 million Blacks. As this pattern continues from the years 2020 to 2065, it effectively removes our people as a viable group within the nation's ethnic tapestry.

An excellent place to close this challenging narrative is to share this quote from the noted scholar and historian, W.E.B. DuBois:

It is doubtful if there is another group of 12 million people in the midst of a modern cultured land who are so widely inhibited and mentally confined as the American Negro.

Within the colored race the philosophy of salvation has by the pressure of caste been curiously twisted and distorted.

Shall they use the torch and dynamite? Shall they go North, or fight it out in the South? Shall they segregate themselves even more than they are now, in states, towns, cities or sections? Shall they leave the country? Are they Americans or foreigners? Shall they stand and sing 'My Country 'Tis of Thee'?

Shall they marry and rear children and save and buy homes, or deliberately commit race suicide?[39]

"What became of the people of Sumer? They perished because they forgot their history." – Goes the ancient riddle

---

[39] BLACK RECONSTRUCTION by W.E.B. Du Bois, 1935

A Daily Protocol for Bio-Integrity

21 Steps, Habits, Instructions

It is often said that "Those who fail to plan, plan to fail." It would be difficult to argue against the rationale of such a belief. In my experience, those times of my life when I drifted along without firmly established goals and targets for daily behavior, have been much less productive.

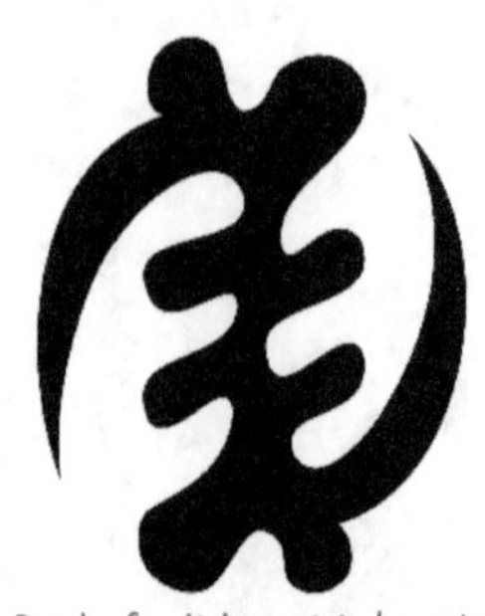

Sankofa: it is not taboo to fetch what is at risk of being left behind.

As I mature through older stages of life, I perceive the profound wisdom of keeping plans, schedules, action lists, daily activities, and journals of the sustainable progress that I am determined to manifest. I AM "the master of my fate" and "I am the captain of my soul," to repeat the famous quote from William Ernest Henley, in his epic poem *Invictus*.

To the **Big Up Manhood,** I offer the following extensive list of constant, daily activities that you should develop into natural habits. I assure that these strategies will add value to your life.

1. **Set and Get Your Goals** – We must always follow some manner of plan for Life, otherwise, we run the danger of drifting along, reacting to whatever surprises that are placed within our attention. Creating a strategic plan helps to consolidate our primary mission and cement our accomplishments throughout a lifetime.

2. **The Nature of a Man** – All aspects of nature and biology are prime areas for study and mastery. Therefore, our male biological

Except God, A symbol expressing the omnipotence of God

functioning must be studied, comprehended, and established as a ruling foundation of how we are to organize our behaviors and habits. Much of what we have seen become normalized within these degenerate societies is contrary to natural order. We must take responsibility for getting it right, least we should suffer terribly for our ignorance.

3. **Use Supplements for Hyper-Nutrition** – One can use a variety of vitamins, minerals, herbs, extracts, and formulas that support male hormonal health, and enhance a man's physical and sexual performance. Many of these supplements are natural balancing compounds found in *adaptogens*, a group of plant compounds that serve to balance glandular functioning.

4. **Exercise Supports Vitality and Longevity** – The many benefits of cardiovascular, strength, and balance exercises are so numerous that they require entire volumes to completely detail. Therefore, to say that these are critically important for men's bio-integrity is easily understood. A recent Harvard University study, published this week, demonstrates the link between men's physical work of heavy lifting with a 44% increase in sperm count compared to more sedentary workers. The same study noted a 42% *reduction* in sperm count between the years 2000 and 2017 among "men seeking fertility treatment."[40]

5. **The Revitalized Man Is On a Worldly Mission** – The world Is mine to mine (as in gold mine). There is immeasurable wealth and resource all across this planet. Much of this

---

[40] PHYSICALLY DEMANDING WORK TIED TO MALE FERTILITY, by Miles Martin, Brigham and Women's Research, Feb 23 2023

abundance is the providence of Nature. There is as well the collected knowledge and wisdom of society. With the right attitude, I can learn and master a vast set of skills, cultivate personal achievements across multiple fields, and share life experiences with the wisest people across multiple civilizations. With all this resource available, there is nothing to keep me from greatness and achievement.

6. **Erectile Dysfunction Is a Symptom of Life Disorder** – A man's ability to maintain a proper hard-on is a strong metaphor for his roles in life. The elaborate mechanism of men's reproductive functioning has so many parallels in the broader society. The integrity of blood flowing through unconstrained veins, combines with the richness of his mental functioning, and serves the appropriateness of his intention. All of these work in perfect harmony with Natural Order to support the penultimate outcome – that of creation of Life. Erectile dysfunction should thus be looked upon as a vital symptom that one's *entire being* is out of balance.

7. **Combatting Cardiovascular Disease (CVD)** – We reasonably conclude that weaknesses of the heart are the consequence of malnutrition and metabolic disorders. The Standard American Diet, which has its subcultural parallel in "Soul Food," is notorious for being high caloric, low nutrition, excessively fatty, and incompatible with our physiological functioning. Meat, dairy, eggs, processed foods, excessive sugar and salt, and chemicals masquerading as food all contribute to the gross persistence of premature death from cardiovascular diseases. We can certainly do better but CVD remains the top killer of people whose bodies are out of shape.

8. **Premature aging & related disorders** – Metabolic disorders, cardiovascular disease, overweight and obesity, arthritis, skinny fat, diabetes, kidney failure, chronic inflammatory conditions, digestive and auto immune disorders, these are all examples of geriatric diseases. This age-related category of disorders also includes ED and prostate hyperplasia. Based upon a number of recent death announcements, we have to wonder why are so many of the hip-hop celebrities dying before reaching 55 years of age? Is it due to *enervation* (an unusual depletion of vital energy due to lifestyle practices)?

9. **Combatting Overweight** – We will often point out how inappropriate the common dietary culture we are born into is. Part of this is due to the excessive feminizing hormones that contaminate the food chain and compromise our hormonal integrity. Beyond a simple formula of calories in/calories out, retaining excess weight indicates that the body's nutrition regulation system detects that we are *starving* for the proper nutrients that comprise our life matrix. When we get the right balance of the eight essential classes of nutrients, we can then maintain the most efficient weight for optimized functioning of the mechanical body.

10. **Overcoming Energy Deficits** – Motivation, inspiration, vitality, response-ability, direct and unhesitating commitment – All these projections of our creative engagement are the consequence of our body's energy generation systems. Optimized energy management of the holistic body is also key to the premier functioning of each of the seventeen body systems. Energy drives brain power, muscular function, immunity, cardiovascular and pulmonary

functioning, etc. The basic formula for energy is a combination of fuel (mainly in the form of glucose, glycogen, and ketones derived from fat cells), along with oxygen, and triggered by metabolic enzymatic processes. Inside every living cell for oxygen-dependent species is an organelle called the *mitochondria*. This is ideally where energy formation takes place. While it might take an extended moment to explain how our energy is converted from food to the cell-activating *adenosine triphosphate*, we know for certain that this process has a logical functioning pathway. It is important to understand the processes and live accordingly because, without energy, we are dead.

11. **Superman Yourself** – Bob Marley, the Prophet, sang about "So much trouble in the world… All you got to do is give a little." His song was not so much a lamentation of the abuse of power that causes the common people to suffer. It was intended to motivate us to actions that combat persisting problems of oppression, exploitation, and other abuses of power. The ***Big Up Manhood*** is called forward to engage at the highest possible level of successful resistance and liberation. To do so, we must maximize all performance factors that give us strength and power. Mind, body, spirit, and mission all come together under our purposeful direction to unleash a heightened level of human performance and the manifestation of willpower.

12. **Don't do like the Romans do**. "Don't swerve; don't lose your nerve." The Romans built one of the most powerful empires in civilization history and then let it collapse due to their decadence, failure to prevent lead toxicity from erasing their collective intelligence, falling under the despotic rule of a bunch of hyperaggressive elitist and

feminized sissies in the Vatican to dominate their social, political, and economic affairs. As well, the Romans abused the authority that providence had afforded them. Ultimately, their degenerate behaviors caused them to lose everything many of their predecessors had fought for centuries.

13. **The Right Diet for an Alpha Male** – For all species, the strongest males are reinforced by the right foods. Their diet is not contaminated with feminizing hormones or endocrine-disrupting chemicals; it is not *sissy food*. Instead, it supports energy formation, hormonal integrity, and a healthy digestive environment, facilitating continuous detoxification. It is hard, if not impossible, for an Alpha Male to maintain his power while suffering from cardiovascular diseases, cancer, obesity, and one or more metabolic diseases. The *optimized* diet for **the Big Up Man** is plant-based, organic, fresh, and homegrown.

14. **Living Superfood Reverses Symptoms of Aging** – WHAT IF you discovered the source of the fabled *Fountain of Youth* and verified that its waters, when consumed, indeed reversed the advance of aging and degeneration? I have been doing my best to confirm to whoever would listen that we have discovered a source of extraordinary youthfulness, vitality, disease resistance, and superior bio-integrity. The greatest challenge is convincing people who have been misinformed all their lives to adhering to a cultural dietary alignment that robs them of their natural birthright of a long and healthy lifespan. We have verified this wisdom of Living Superfood. It works, so how do we convince many more people to take advantage of what has been proven? WHAT IF you knew this too?

15. **Combatting Prostate Diseases** – It is widely believed that American men, particularly Afri-Amer men, are at great risk of developing and dying from prostate cancer. Well, there is a lot of misinformation and propaganda from the profiteers in the healthcare industry that is driving our misunderstandings. I have researched this field for decades and have made several shocking pronouncements based on what I have confirmed. These include:

- Cancer is a relatively new disease in the evolution of humanity and has exploded in incidence over the past 125 years, from 1900 to 2021, expanding from a rate of 1-in-24 to 2-in-5, even as funding for cancer research has increased unabated. The National Cancer Institute (NCI), estimates that in the United States, approximately 39.5% of men and women will be diagnosed with cancer at some point during their lifetime based on 2017-2019 data. This estimate is based on current incidence rates and may vary depending on various factors such as age, sex, and race/ethnicity;

- Prostate cancer, while receiving a lot of promotion, is generally not a large cause of mortality without the toxicity of aggressive traditional cancer treatments of radiation, surgery, and chemotherapies that inhibit natural cell replication;

- The standard test for *prostate-specific antigen* (PSA) is not what it claims to be – a test for prostate cancer;

- Dr. Richard Ablin, universally acknowledged as the scientist to identify PSA, is one of the most vocal critics of widespread testing using his discovery. In his book **THE GREAT PROSTATE HOAX: *How Big Medicine Hijacked***

the PSA Test and Caused a Public Health Disaster, he exposes the many pathways by which men are deceived by how "the emerging biotech industry and the urology community focused their collective energies on an irresistible financial opportunity: 30 million age-appropriate American men" for exploitation using the fear of cancer as a campaign that he likens to that of the military;

- As bizarre a twist as could be imagined, increased numbers of men, disproportionately Blacks, are being told that their prostate disease is a consequence of too much testosterone and subsequently being treated with estrogen hormone therapies. This is the same process administered to sexual deviants forced by the state to undergo *chemical castration*;

- Over the 30 years since I have been aware of this public health catastrophe, it has been one great frustration trying to set my Black Brothers straight on the facts about this grand deception. But, on the contrary, it seems like every new diagnosis among Afri-Amer men of prostate diseases serves to initiate additional volunteers from our community to advocate for the aggressive campaign;

- In truth, increasing diagnoses of reproductive disease in men and women are tied to the *western diet* that is overly heavy on consuming meat, highly processed food, and estrogen-contaminated dairy products (which are logically incompatible with our diet – what other species consumes the milk of another species, especially after weaning?)

- Here's a simple question: <u>Got milk, got prostate disease?</u>

16. **Mastering the Breath** – We talked earlier about energy formation and how that process drives all of our body's life systems. Fuel, oxygen, and metabolic enzyme function are at the heart of energy formation. For this formula to function at its highest capacity, the integrity of respiration must be prioritized. In addition, the highest-quality breathing is key to other body processes beyond mere energy production. These include avoiding adrenal fatigue (overstressing the fight or flight hormone functioning), lowering blood pressure, maximizing brain functioning, preventing cancer, opening up blood flow throughout the body, reducing metabolic diseases, and avoiding premature aging. Advanced breathing techniques are a proven way to summon immediate strength and stamina. (200 push-ups, anyone?)

17. **Drug Free Temperance** – For the **Big Up Man** to enjoy his optimal physical condition, he is best to avoid consuming alcohol and smoking marijuana. This temperance should be sustained for many life-enhancing reasons. Here I am referring to specific reproductive advantages for sperm integrity, Increasing sperm count, and preserving male fertility. We have long been aware of the evidence that alcoholic beverages negatively impact fertility in experiments on lab rats. At the time that I was writing about this research, it was obvious that our reproductive males of the hip-hop generation were the "lab rats" for the dangerous malt liquor industry. The long-term impact to these men was devastating; we are currently witnessing them dying by their 40s to 50s from diseases regarded as affecting primarily older people. My research on the contamination of reefer supplies that were distributed

among the inner-city residents showed that at one point in the mid-1990s, as much as 75% of these showed evidence of fungus contamination, a sure recipe for immune compromise and acute pulmonary infections. For these and so many other justifications, we would be best to give up indulging in these self-limiting and self-destructive lifestyle habits until a different time when we can ensure their safety. For me, there is no space for alcohol, although I do believe that herbal, *medicinal* marijuana has value.

18. **Strength and Stamina Beyond Belief** – I am relishing this lifestyle I'm describing in the pages of this book regarding the **Big Up Manhood** paradigm shift. You should be able to sense the enthusiasm that I bring to these topics. I hope you are informed, inspired, and excited to learn these many life-enhancing practices, strategies, and tactics for obtaining and retaining superior health. I often (perhaps *too often*) boast about my daily push-up routine. At age 67 years, five months, and 11 days, completing 57 consecutive days of 200 or more push-ups in a single set for my first set of the day seems miraculous. I am immensely proud to make such a boast; I hope you tolerate me for this. In addition, I set a new lifetime record for cumulative push-ups in a single day during this period – 1800 total. That caused a bit of a strain, and I've since dropped down from averaging 700-1200 a day to an even 500, which I am trying to do in just three sets. My strength and stamina are spectacular in many other daily activities. I am living proof that being a senior citizen can also be incredibly athletic.

19. **Exogenous Feminizing Hormones Impact the Male Brain** – We acknowledge the distinctions between male and female brain structures and subtle hormonal differences. As well it

is proven that when this happens to a fetus undergoing sexual differentiation during the first months after conception, this can lead to three biomarkers of "gender ambiguity." How does excessive exposure to feminizing hormones (exogenous estrogens) compromise a man's brain, mind, and body?:

- Reduced libido and sexual function due to low testosterone production;

- Cognitive impairment, including decreased attention, memory, and executive function;

- Depression and anxiety due to elevated estrogen levels;

- Reduced muscle mass and strength;

- Increased risk of cardiovascular disease, including heart attack and stroke.

20. **Rebuilding Your Manhood Roles** – In fatherhood, family and community, and as a contributor to the nation and the world, maturing to responsible adult manhood comes with challenging and demanding responsibilities. A common "Red Pill" meme has become widely quoted and states, "Hard times create strong men. Strong men create good times. Good times create weak men. And weak men create hard times."[41] Unfortunately, these times are seeing a proliferation of soft males, weaklings, and sissified roles across societal institutions. This is unsustainable, and we must change that equation for our group's survival and sustainable development.

---

[41] Those Who Remain: A Postapocalyptic Novel, by G. Michael Hopf, 2016

21. **Old Habits Die Hard; New Habits Form Quickly** – There can be no half-stepping, to establish a paradigm-shifting habitual transformation. You know what you intended when you set upon this pathway. Don't swerve. Don't lose your nerve. If you fall, pick yourself up, dust yourself off, and start over again. You need and deserve a major victory in life; this is where it will be extracted.

As we work to overcome a myriad of challenges to our essential manhood, we must never forget timeless insights and instructions from sages like Bob Marley, who we should regard as a prophet for our generations:

You see men sailing on their ego trip
Blast off on their spaceship
Million miles from reality
No care for you, no care for me
So much trouble in the world
So much trouble in the world
All you got to do is give a little

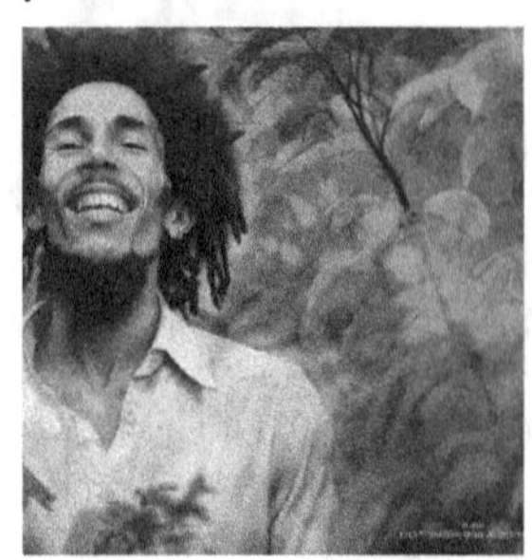

Now they sitting on a time bomb
Now I know the time has come
What goes on up is coming on down
Goes around and comes around
So much trouble in the world
So much trouble in the world
All you got to do is give a little
Give a little

Big Up Manhood Sexual Power
What Is (Not) Up with Erectile Dysfunction?

"A woman simply is, but a man must become. Masculinity is risky and elusive. It is achieved by a revolt from woman, and it confirmed only by other men. Manhood coerced into sensitivity is no manhood at all." – Camille Paglia

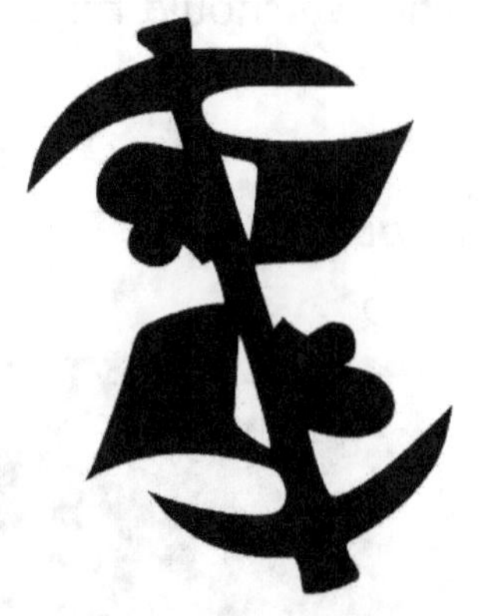

Okuafo Pa represents diligence, hard work, and entrepreneurship, all characteristic of a successful farmer

Today let's focus on men's issues and how to keep your "man stuff" going strong. Unfortunately, this is a conversation that men have too infrequently, especially considering the steadily rising incidences of men's fertility problems and reproductive disorders.

While women are stronger at "showing up" regarding health maintenance issues, men must also improve their focus. On average, within all ethnic groups and across the world of nations, women are outliving men.

Men's hormonal changes throughout life have a profound impact on overall health. We remember those years in our late teens and early adulthood when we convinced ourselves we were invincible. We could outwork other men around us, lift heavier weights, run further distances, stay up past midnight, and still manage to bounce up early that day to return to the workplace. During that phase of our lives, we would eat anything (or believed that we could), and it did not negatively impact our strength and vitality.

In our lifetime, this idea that we could do and eat anything and still maintain youthful integrity has changed significantly. The modern food supply has numerous components which undermine men's hormonal integrity. A large class of contaminants in food and commonly-used substances have been called "endocrine-disrupting chemicals." Abbreviated as EDCs, these have been causing havoc with hormonal integrity since biological chemists first identified them in the mid-20th Century.

Many of these EDCs mimic or disrupt the action of a set of primary female hormones called estrogens. So what happens to a man when estrogen-mimicking disruptors throw off his natural hormonal balance? Negative effects can range from increased incidence of prostate diseases, especially prostate cancer, rising risk of various forms of cancer, loss of drive, erectile dysfunction, and even the growth of "man boobs," also known as enlarged breasts in men or gynecomastia.

The shocking rise in prostate disease diagnoses should be of grave concern to men. Fortunately, the causes of these diseases, which can range from inflammatory swelling to cancer, have been identified and are thus largely preventable. The national drive toward PSA testing among men undoubtedly plays a significant role in the increase in diagnoses we see. However, prostate antigen testing has not been without controversy. Even the discoverer of PSA, Dr. Richard Ablin, has stated his opposition to how the exploitation of his discovery has proceeded. His book, ***THE GREAT PROSTATE HOAX: How Big Medicine Hijacked the PSA Test and Caused a Public***

Health Disaster, is a scathing indictment of the medical profession, PSA testing, and the risky treatments that have become popularized.

Our strategies should focus on avoiding the conditions which give rise to reproductive disorders, inflammatory diseases, and other factors which advance aging processes. Reinforcing youthful levels of androgen hormones, the primary of which is free testosterone is one of our nutritional strategies for keeping that "man stuff" vibrant for an extended lifespan and quality of life.

Here are just a few simple steps that help keep the "upful" man in **Big Up Manhood**.

- Avoid hormone-disrupting chemicals in the food and environment. These include female hormones in dairy products and milk fat, hormones added to animal feed to increase the rate at which feeder animals gain weight, and a vast spectrum of chemicals identified as EDCs.

- Use supplements to reinforce your hormonal integrity. Two particular favorites of mine, which are a part of the anti-aging supplements I cover in ***LIVING SUPERFOOD LONGEVITY***, are stinging nettle extract, which increases circulating free testosterone, and bioidentical pregnenolone, which serves as a nutritional precursor to hormone synthesis within the glandular system. Other powerful supplements supporting prostate health include saw palmetto, zinc, and ginger.

- Mix a proper balance of the three types of exercise. In support of anti-aging strategies, I recommend that we all engage in cardiovascular exercise, including sports and running, strength training using weights or gravity resistance, and balance exercises like yoga, Tai Chi, or Qi Gong.

On average, life expectancy for men is less than that of women, but it need not be so. We can significantly extend our average lifespan with the right daily habits and lifestyle priorities. There is a great reason to be optimistic to all the men who will listen. Apply the principles you are learning during the 21-day workshop to live long, love strong, and prosper.

The Causes and Effects of Low-T

What are the signs, causes, symptoms, and treatments for low testosterone, also known as "Low-T?" In how many ways does this primary male hormone impact our physical well-being, disease resistance, strength, and motivation? Are we witnessing a significant decline in male fertility, energy, power, and drive in our modern societies?

These important questions need satisfactory answers, and we intend to respond to them to your satisfaction. Therefore, I have gathered years of research and verified that they are effective with my hands-on investigation and experimentation. People are constantly amazed at my youthful physiology, demonstrable strength and endurance, and ability to resist diseases. I must reveal that it's not superior genetics or expensive medicine that is my success formula. What I have tapped into is a spectrum of natural science-based strategies that have allowed me to reverse the aging process and get my manhood on track to support my happiness well into my senior years.

This **Big Up Manhood 21-Day Protocol** will unquestionably show you a new direction to avoid hormonal degradation due to neglect, a bad diet, and engaging in futile remedies that don't hit their mark. You need to hit the bullseye every time and feel confident that you have access to the full level of male performance that you knew when you were decades younger. Your physical status must command respect from men and women alike. It would help if you were all you could to protect your family, community, and everything you truly cherish. Big Up, Man. Much Respect!

Safe Supplements for the Big Up Man

At this point, I want to expound further on the spectrum of youthful androgen hormone supplements. I don't just want to make a long list of the nutrients I use but also briefly explain exactly what they should be expected to do for you.

22 Powerful Male Restoration Supplements

1. **Bioavailable Folate** – (Folic Acid; Vitamin B9) – This is the natural form of the water-soluble vitamin B9 found in many foods. It is critical for forming D.N.A. and R.N.A. as it is involved in protein metabolism. In addition, it plays a key role in breaking down the stress hormone homocysteine, which is important for cell growth and metabolism is needed to produce healthy red blood cells, and supplementation is used to treat deficiencies, certain types of anemia, and other problems in people with digestive issues, kidney or liver disease, or alcohol abuse.

2. **Fenugreek Seeds** – This nutritional powerhouse has a long record of benefits for men's hormonal health. Reported benefits for men include increasing libido and sex drive, overcoming erectile dysfunction (E.D.), increasing sperm count and mobility, increasing the blood level of free

testosterone, helping to prevent hair loss, and as a nutritional aid for bodybuilding. Additional benefits are that it helps with digestion, reduces constipation, and balances cholesterol levels. I consume ground fenugreek seeds every day.

3. **Bioidentical Pregnenolone** – A hormonal precursor needed to feed glandular functioning and hormonal integrity, cultivated from wild yams (*Dioscorea villosa*). An endogenous steroid is important for the biosynthesis of most steroidal hormones manufactured by the body. The hormones are particularly helpful to reproductive functioning and include androgens, estrogens, progestogens (facilitate childbearing), glucocorticoids, neurosteroids, and mineralocorticoids.

4. **Stinging Nettle Extract** – This commonly found herb is noted for its potential to rebalance a man's youthful testosterone. As we age, our ability to produce hormones associated with reproduction naturally declines. Among men (and, to a lesser extent, women as well), a decline in free testosterone is associated with male prostate problems, can contribute to muscle wasting, and speeds up aging processes among both sexes. One of the strategies that one can use to prevent this is using the Stinging Nettle Extract supplement, which not only helps to "prevent the binding of sex hormone-binding globulin to testosterone," which will allow more free testosterone to circulate, but these lignans also nutritionally reinforce the base of amino acids which provide material for the manufacture of hormones.

5. **Men's Passion Booster** – This formula provides high-performance support for active men. It features ingredients such as Tongkat Ali (botanical name, *Eurycoma longifolia*, also known as "Ali's walking stick" or "Longjack"), used traditionally for centuries as a natural remedy for fatigue and sexual health. Other components include Vitamin B6, amino acids L-Arginine and L-Citruline, oat straw extract, and Tribulus Extract. Each of these ingredients has been studied for their benefits in combatting erectile dysfunction, improving circulation, antioxidant and antibacterial, boosting immunity and fever reduction, mood enhancement, relieving anxiety, reducing symptoms of depression, improving cognitive and brain function, aiding in hemoglobin production, rich in minerals, cancer prevention, eye health support, improved exercise tolerance, combatting high blood pressure, aiding against peripheral arterial disease, and increasing exercise capacity.

6. **Saw Palmetto** – Of undeniable concern among aging men are issues related to prostate health, the effects of shifting hormone levels affected by aging, and environmental stresses from endocrine-disrupting chemicals we constantly encounter. Among the challenges men face are rising incidences of benign prostatic hypertrophy (BPH), which affects many men from the age of 40 and can result in moderate-to-severe lower urinary tract symptoms that impact one's quality of life. Another great concern is the rising incidence of prostate cancer among men, especially within the most developed countries. Numerous benefits of the herbal supplement saw palmetto include modulating hormonal effects, preventing hair loss, the positive impact of zinc supplementation (zinc is a major component of the

herb), combating or preventing inflammatory conditions in the reproductive tract, and it is a powerful agent for strategies to rejuvenate one's hormonal balance. In addition, for women as well as men, supplementation with this herb is associated with increased libido. For women, the suggested daily dose of 160 mg is half of that recommended for men, ranging from 160-320 mg daily.

7. **Ginger Root Powder** – Most of us know about the awesome benefits of consuming fresh ginger root juice daily. As a supplement in its powdered form, it brings many great benefits. These include one of the top antioxidant, anti-inflammatory nutritional superfoods, cancer prevention, and treatment, promotes digestion, improves cardiovascular function, combats metabolic disorders, helps to maintain optimal weight, anti-arthritic, helps balance blood lipids, and helps to preserve and improve cognitive functioning as we age. Ginger is one of four nutritional herbs we should consume daily, along with cinnamon, cayenne, and turmeric.

8. **DHEA (Dehydroepiandrosterone)** – DHEA is a hormone naturally produced by the adrenal glands and involved in "more than 150 metabolic functions". It is a fact that DHEA levels begin to decline after age thirty, leading to aging symptoms such as sluggishness, weight gain, and lowered libido. Therefore supplementation with this natural steroid hormone becomes a critical component of any anti-aging nutrition program. The many benefits attributed to DHEA include boosting immune function, combatting adrenal fatigue, depression, obesity, helping to prevent dangerous visceral fat, osteoporosis, muscle strength, sex hormone functioning, reproductive health issues such as menopause,

vaginal atrophy, erectile dysfunction, along with psychological conditions, cognitive functioning, Alzheimer's, combatting cardiovascular diseases, is important to male testes functioning, combats osteoporosis, and its use by athletes and bodybuilders for building lean muscle mass, preventing fat accumulation. Because of the impact of DHEA on athletic performance, sports associations have added it to their banned lists.

9. **Ashwagandha Extract** – *Withania somnifera*, known commonly as ashwagandha or winter cherry, is an evergreen shrub in the Solanaceae or nightshade family that grows in India, the Middle East, and parts of Africa. It is one of the widely researched adaptogens. The benefits of ashwagandha include better cardiovascular performance, improved sleep, combatting adrenal fatigue, improved brain functioning, concentration and memory, helps to relieve depression, stress and anxiety, counters infertility, anti-inflammatory immune-booster, helps to reduce blood sugar levels, increased testosterone levels, increased fertility, increases sperm production, an aid to athletic performance and strength, and is a natural aphrodisiac. Cautions regarding ashwagandha include side effects like upset stomach, diarrhea, vomiting, and possible interaction with pharmaceutical medications. It is not recommended for pregnant and breastfeeding women, and it is preferred that you take periodic breaks from using it continuously.

10. **Zinc Picolinate** – Zinc has been referred to as "the ultimate sex mineral" by a men's health magazine because of its impact on fertility, potency, and overall sexual health. Those who faithfully use this supplement do so for good reasons, such as facilitating sperm production and motility,

boosting levels of free testosterone, resisting or reversing prostate diseases such as *benign prostatic hyperplasia* (BPH) and *prostatitis*, boosting immunity, reducing damage from alcoholic liver disease, preventing thyroid glandular disease, and cellular repair.

11. **Vitamin D3** – This important nutrient is part of a group of fat-soluble components that increase nutrient absorption of minerals key to metabolic function. Its spectrum of benefits includes strengthening bones and teeth, supporting immune system function, anti-inflammatory, balancing androgen hormones, combatting erectile dysfunction, facilitating sperm production, muscular growth, hair retention, and weight loss, as it also is reported to support mental health. The Vitamin D group is often called "the sun vitamin" because your body produces this hormone-like substance when exposed to 20 minutes of sunshine on the skin each day.

12. **Tongkat Ali** – This amazing herb has a long record of use as a natural sexual stimulant in men and women. Other benefits include boosting energy, revitalization, muscle development, stress relief, increasing testosterone production, aiding libido and sexual appetite, strengthening muscular and skeletal systems, supporting weight optimization, enhancing immunity, known anti-cancer properties, strengthening bones and teeth, improving mental balance, combatting metabolic diseases, antibacterial and anti-parasitic, and its anti-ulcer potential.

13. **Vitamin B-complex** contains all eight fat-soluble B vitamins in one pill. These include:

- B1 (thiamine) – Serves an essential role in metabolism and converting nutrients into energy.

- B2 (riboflavin) – Helps convert food into energy and is an antioxidant.

- B3 (niacin) – Involved in DNA production and repair, metabolism, and cellular signaling.

- B5 (pantothenic acid) – This also assists in energy conversion along with hormone and cholesterol production.

- B6 (pyridoxine) – This critically important vitamin is involved in amino acid metabolism and creating red blood cells and neurotransmitters.

- B7 (biotin) – This vitamin helps metabolize carbohydrates and fats and regulates gene expression.

- B9 (folate) – This essential vitamin is critical to cell growth, amino acid metabolism, cell formation, and dividing red and white blood cells.

- B12 (cobalamin) – Often called to caution due to a need for vegans to supplement, B12 is essential for neurological formation, DNA production, and regulating red blood cell development. It is found in vegan sources such as sea vegetables, nutritional yeast, and supplements.

14. **Black Maca** - Maca is a Peruvian plant grown in the Andes mountains. It is a cruciferous vegetable, meaning that it is related to broccoli, cabbage, and kale. Maca is a common ingredient in Peruvian cooking that gives dishes an earthy flavor. Maca root plant can be ground into powder and

added to meals or smoothies. Aside from its culinary uses, maca may also have several health benefits

15. **Tribulus Terrestris Extract** (fruit) - A powerful sexual tonic, Tribulus tops the charts of herbal Viagra. Studies have shown that this herb elevates the luteinizing hormone (LH), increasing free testosterone levels in healthy males. This, in turn, will increase sexual desire, libido, and improve the quality of sperm while making it more nimble; in some cases, it will help to remedy erectile dysfunction, and it has proven to be helpful in cases of premature ejaculation. One of the main compounds of this herb is a phytochemical known as "protodioscin," with one study showing it helps to boost nitric oxide production. Nitric Oxide is an essential element of an erection, enabling the smooth muscles of the penis to relax, allowing uninterrupted blood to flow to this area. Tribulus will stimulate the production of sex hormones without affecting other bodily systems.

16. **Horny Goat Weed** (Epimedium sagittatum) Extract - Horny goat weed is an herbal supplement that some people use as a kind of "natural Viagra" to treat erectile dysfunction. Some studies suggest it has other positive effects, especially on bone health. However, more rigorous human clinical studies are needed to clarify the health benefits of horny goat weed. Caution should be taken if you have certain medical conditions or take certain medications. Consult your healthcare provider to determine if a horny goat weed supplement is right for you.

17. **Fadogia Agrestis Extract** - Fadogia agrestis is a plant native to Nigeria. The stem of this plant is used to make medicines. It is a well-known plant due to its ability to increase the

production of the male hormone testosterone and enhance sexual desire. But this plant can also provide many other benefits due to its presence of antioxidants and some plant compounds. Not only this, but Fadogia agrestis also works as a natural supplement to prevent the accumulation of excess fat in the body and also makes the person fit by burning fat.

18. **Pomegranate Peel Extract** - Pomegranates grow in many countries because of their ability to stand the heat and cold, decorative value, industrial usefulness, and, more importantly, health-giving properties. The health benefits of pomegranate peels might even inspire you to start eating them, not to mention that they taste good!

19. **Cacao Seed Extract** (Theobroma cacao) - The health benefits of cacoa (cocoa) include decreased inflammation, improved heart and brain health, blood sugar and weight control, and healthy teeth and skin. It's nutritious and easy to add to your diet in creative ways. However, use non-alkalized cocoa powder or dark chocolate containing more than 70% cocoa to maximize health benefits. Remember that chocolate still contains significant quantities of sugar and fats, so if you use it, stick to reasonable portion sizes and combine it with a healthy balanced diet.

20. **Luteolin Extract** (Japanese sophora flower) - Sophora japonica Extract is extracted from dried flower buds of the legume Sophora japonica L. The main active ingredient is rutin. Sophora extract has the functions of anti-oxidation, inhibition of cancer cells, and protection of nerve cells. Sophora japonica is a commonly used Chinese medicine. It is a dried flower bud of the leguminous plant Huai, tastes

bitter and slightly cold, and has the effects of cooling blood to stop bleeding, clearing the liver, and reducing fire. In recent years, domestic and foreign medical workers have researched its role and found that its active ingredients are anti-cancer and anti-cancer, anti-platelet aggregation, analgesia, antibacterial, antiviral, anti-aging, anti-inflammatory, anti-allergy, anti-free radical and anti-oxidation A variety of activities, such as improving myocardial circulation, clearing heat and detoxifying, lowering blood lipids, softening blood vessels, anti-inflammatory and nourishing kidney, etc., have non-toxic, harmless, non-lethal, carcinogenic, teratogenic (causing developmental malformations), and mutagenic effects.

21. **D.I.M.** (Diindolylmethane) - 3,3 diindolylmethane (D.I.M.) is a major digestive product that is found naturally in the Brassica (mustard) family of vegetables such as cabbage, brussels sprouts, and broccoli. D.I.M. has been extensively studied for decades by various research groups. It boasts several rejuvenating properties, such as D.N.A. repair, anti-tumor, and anti-viral effects. Crucially, D.I.M. is also capable of regulating the sex hormones in the body… In addition, D.I.M. has been shown to inhibit prostate cells from progressing from one growth phase to another. This effect has been extensively studied in esophageal, colorectal, breast, endometrial, oral, and prostate cancer.

22. **Black Pepper Extract** - Black pepper extract or piperine has the potential to provide numerous health benefits, according to research. Studies have shown that it contains anti-inflammatory, anticancer, and antimicrobial abilities and its bioavailability quality, which may boost the absorption of certain nutrients, including vitamins,

minerals, and phytochemical molecules, by our digestive system. This works particularly well with compounds such as curcumin/ turmeric, which provide their own excellent health benefits. Piperine may also enhance the absorption of certain medications. Since there is no FDA/ standard dosage for consuming black pepper extract supplements, always get accurate medical information and permission before ingesting any product.

23. **Test X180 Boost** Formula – Force Factor™, the manufacturer of a supplement I use, claims that their product "is designed to help support testosterone levels through premium ingredients for increased blood flow, more energy, stamina, endurance, help build lean muscle mass," in addition to increases in the level of free testosterone in the blood, increased sexual performance, aids in boosting athletic performance. They claim it works best combined with traditional male vitality ingredients such as Panax ginseng, cordyceps, and Tribulus Terrestris.

I have used several of this long list of manhood-boosting herbs and supplements for over a decade. While I could go on ad infinitum about the health benefits, unproven claims, possible side effects, cautions, and hearsay about this spectrum of nutritional additives, my *bottom line* is adding herbs, vitamins, supplements, and supplements male enhancements to your diet is cutting-edge science. This stuff delivers for someone like myself who wants every edge and advantage that can be utilized toward longevity, high performance, disease resistance, rapid recovery, and optimized physical form.

Regularly using so many nutritional supplements can get a bit pricey. I don't take each of them every day. I tend to rotate 9-

12 different supplements daily while obtaining the best nutritional spectrum through consuming a maximum of fresh, organic, and locally grown fruits and vegetables as I can maintain. Superfoods are also very important in my ***Furiously Vegan*** strategy to keep the cardiovascular, blood, brain, glandular, and musculoskeletal systems functioning at peak performance – in addition to all of the body's 17 functional systems.

I hope you come to a judgment similar to my own that we must emphasize the need to empower *the whole man*. We Big Up Men will not be reduced to pronouns, as is the case across the conflict about gender dysbiosis and debates about what constitutes a he, she, him, her, it, or a *whatever!.*

We are advocating for the unification of all the parts, be they the physiological representation of sexual organs, glandular system, and brain structure, or those parts of gender identification that relate to an individual's history of psychological experiences, which could be brilliantly empowering or tragically traumatic. Also, the configuration of the social order into which we have been domiciled greatly affects how we judge behaviors that complement our inheritance of feminine and masculine expression. We *hope* to have been born into a nation with a healthy and sustainable reproductive and mental health state.

I've done my best to give you the correct information for your primary masculine development. Take this research to heart to keep the Man in your ***Big Up Manhood***… She'll thank you for it as well.

Affirmations

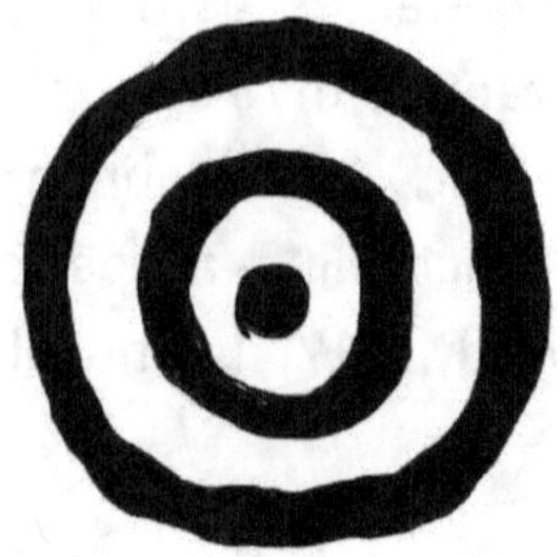

Adinkrahene is the King of the Adinkra symbols, standing for authority, leadership, and charisma

The Alchemist Pledge

I swear before Ra, the almighty force of energy.

I swear before the Great Mother Goddess, Her womb is the source of Life.

I swear before all the mighty forces of nature, the Neteru & Orishas.
I swear before the Great Ancestors, saints, and the martyrs.
I swear before the Wise & Esteemed Elders of my global community.
I swear before all the children, the babies, and their mothers.
I swear before all the brave ones whom we trust to carry the spear.

I pledge before all of My Great Family, who assemble as one, that I am prepared to step up to all of the duties and responsibilities required of me as an Alchemist. I am pledged, in any and all circumstances, to transform that which is dull into that which is brilliant. I am sensitized to every opportunity to confront all challenges and to master over problems that have put all humanity in peril. I WILL move forward to build **STEAMSHIPS** to educate our youth to preeminence through the mastery of all sciences. I WILL redirect the old, enslaving forces of FEAR and PANIC into liberating ideologies that forge a new pathway to sustainable development. I WILL be constant in my creativity, sensitivity, positive alignment, and resourcefulness, all toward forging a new pathway to sustainable development.

I AM the Alchemist - I turn that which is dull into that which is brilliant. I am energized by the Sun, purified and given life by the Waters, grounded in the pristine Earth of my Mother continent, and given wings by the Breath of Life, whose airs project my vision over the horizons.

I AM the Alchemist. I AM at once the past, present, and the future. I AM that I AM.

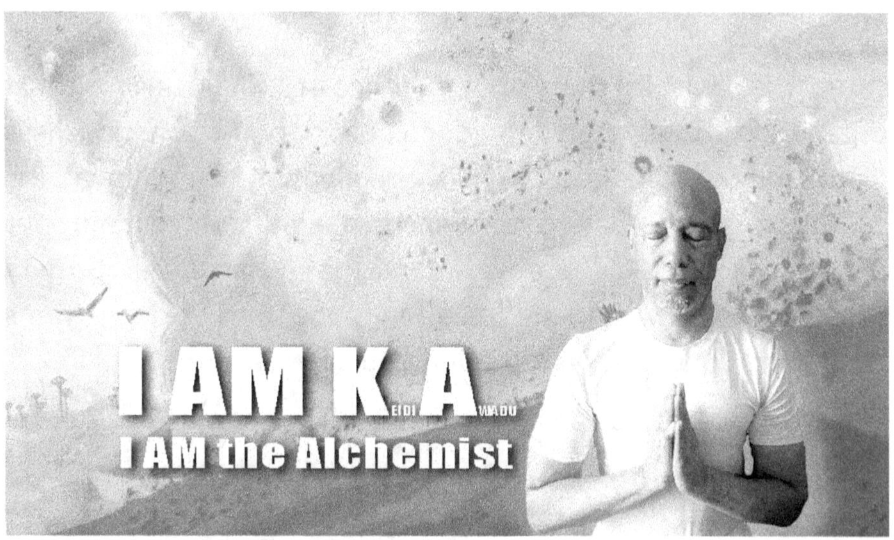

The Ausarian Initiation

Over the 20 years since I launched the webcast network of LIBRadio and LIBtv, I have had the honor and privilege of interviewing many of our generation's greatest minds. This forum centered around Pan-African sustainable development, an Afrocentric pedagogy, and projecting the perspective of world history and political affairs from the minds and viewpoints of African/Black scholarship. Over these decades, our *Living In Black* curriculum consolidated around more than a dozen central themes, including culture, consciousness, historical perspectives, entertainment, economics, education, health, labor, justice, politics, spirituality, family, conflict, Pan-African affairs, future studies, and sustainable development.

Across this broad spectrum, all synchronized into the grand perspective of who Africans are in civilization, we often focused on spiritual traditions to empower our global family. One of my frequent and beloved guests was <u>Dr. Ra Un Nefer Amen, also called the Shekhem Ur Shekhem</u>, who is credited with founding **The Ausar Auset Society** in 1973.

Of many valuable transforming processes that this spiritual organization integrated into our contemporary consciousness were multiple manifestations of initiation into functional spiritual systems that have been recovered from our ancient Nile Valley cultural heritage. Here the Ausar Auset Society describes The Ausarian Initiation, one of the programs conducted under the organization's auspices.

> Of all the spiritual systems that were practiced in Ancient Egypt, the Ausarian Initiation system was the most effective means of leading Man (men and women) to the attainment of divinity, the essence of our being.
>
> Treading the path of Initiation to Divinity awakens and optimizes Man's higher mental abilities, moral nature, talents and spiritual faculties for her /his personal and social benefit, as there is a tendency among people to excuse all of our failings on our humanness, it should be clear that the "human" stage of Man's development represents our spiritual infancy and therefore must be transcended.
>
> Ancient Egypt's great accomplishments in all areas of civilization: women's rights, education, spirituality,

government, and the arts and sciences (mathematics, three scripts, architecture, metallurgy. astronomy, medicine, literature, etc.) were due to the optimization of the talents, intelligence, morality and spirituality of its people. The Ausarian Initiation program will do the same for you.[42]

The full initiation is an ongoing education and guided meditation conducted by the Society through their international collective of local franchises. However, I was never a member of the Society as my course of Kemetic spiritual development took a distinct pathway that led to my May 2012 ordination into *The Sacred Order of the Sons of Ra Ministries* – I AM KheperRa, the keeper of the morning sun, the one that sees over the horizon and ushers in the New Day.

Although I never became a member of the Ausar Auset Society or numerous other Kemet-centric spiritual organizations, it has always been my mission to champion several of these groups' existence, mission, and accomplishments as I became aware of their existence.

To the men of this **Big Up Manhood** rites-of-passage program, it is highly recommended that you explore this pathway of becoming adept at African-centered spiritual comprehension. We will realize our true identities and mission in Life through such a pathway of enlightenment and surrender to our indigenous spiritual roots.

As I wrote in my 1998 book ***CONSPIRACIES AND HIGH CRIMES***:

---

[42] The Ausarian Initiation, extracted from the online site of the Orlando Ausar Auset Society.

"I further solemnly promise and swear that with the divine permission I will from this day forward apply myself unto the Great Work which is so to purify and exalt my spiritual nature, that with the Divine Aid, I may at length attain to be more than Human, and thus gradually raise and unite myself to my Higher and Divine Genius, and that in this event, I will not abuse the great power entrusted unto me."[43]

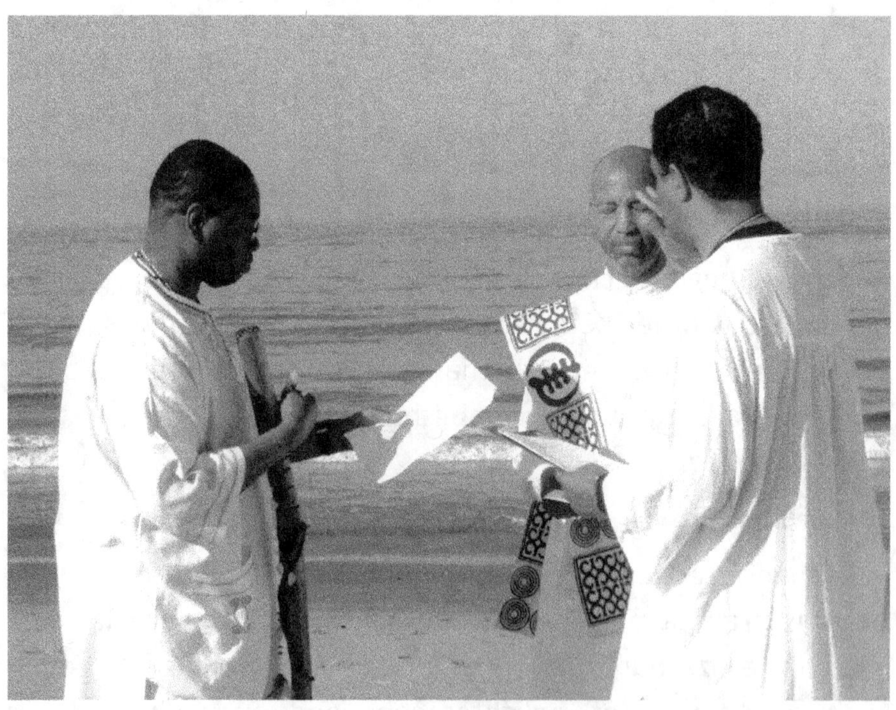

---

[43] The Original Account of the Teachings, Rites and Ceremonies of the Hermetic Order of THE GOLDEN DAWN by Israel Regardie, Llewellyn Publications, 1995, pg. 106

The Ausarian Prayer

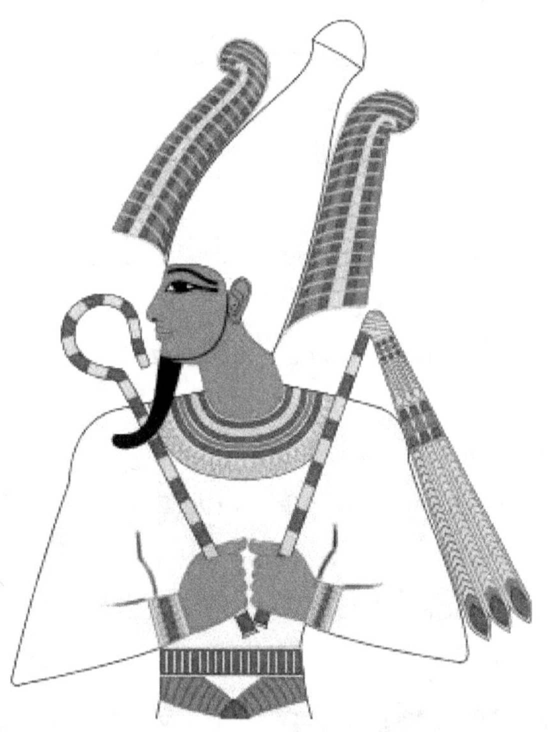

I am black as the night
From which the light of the new day ascends
I am the past, the present, and the future
I am the Anointed of God
I AM That I AM

I am the many blended colors of Life
Which lights the bridge into the New Age
I am the seed, plant, and the flower
I am the Anointed of the Earth
I AM What I AM

Redefining FEAR and PANIC

F.E.A.R. (Is Used to Excite and Control Behaviors)

F - Forward thinking, planning, and acting for the Future

E - Evolving Economic development to Enable sustainability

A - Africa holds the resources to solve the world's problems

R - Restructure existing spending to Repair ourselves

P.A.N.I.C. (Compels a Powerful Sense of URGENCY!)

P - Produce Products and services

A - As Alchemists, it's All in, no half-stepping

N - Nature provides for us the best medicine

I - Investing Intelligently toward Intentional ROI

C - Culture is the vehicle to best Conserve/Consolidate Civilization

Educating Black Youth to African Empowerment

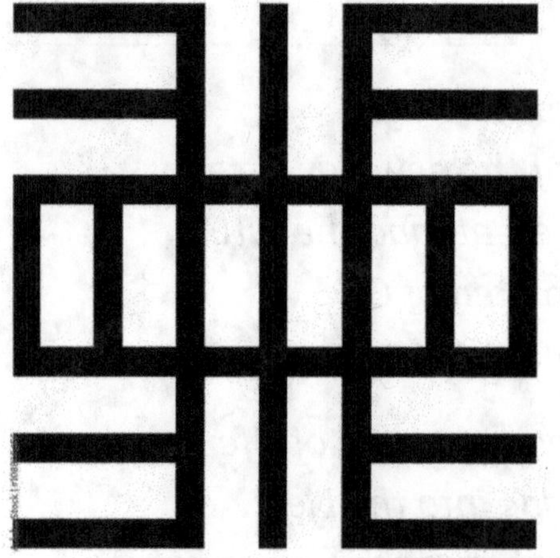

Nea Onnim: "When he who does not know learns, he gets to know." Adinkra symbol of knowledge, life-long education, and a continued quest for knowledge.

STEAMSHIPS Education for African Youth to Power

S - Science

T – Technology

E - Engineering

A - Arts

M - Mathematics

S - Spirituality

H - Holistic Health

I - Innovation

P - Prosperity

S – Sustainability

Conclusion or Beginnings?

To control a people you must first control what they think about themselves and how they regard their history and culture. And when your conqueror makes you ashamed of your culture and your history, he needs no prison walls and no chains to hold you. – Dr. John Henrick Clarke

We have taken many turns over the course of examining the problems and challenges facing ours and future generations.

I have tried to highlight the complexity of manhood as it has evolved over the last century.

My personal observations during this two-thirds of a century have spanned many key facets of our successes and failures

We are faced at this time with an urgent existential set of crises that will determine the fate of a 21 generation legacy of our existence as captives within a foreign and frequently hostile culture.

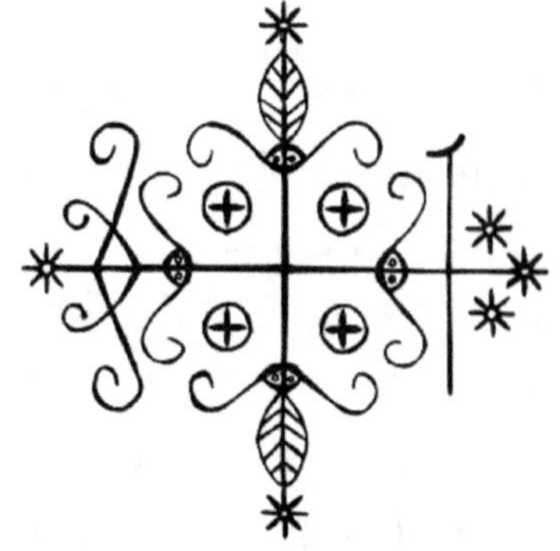

LEGBA: West African and Caribbean Voodoo symbol signifies Legba's control over communications and forms of passage.

As the Jamaican Poet Laureate Mutabaruka chanted, "It nuh good fi stay inna white man country too long."

We are at the crossroads of our long Maafa journey. The decisive moves made on behalf of our large ethnic group during the next 45 years will largely decide our fate.

As has often been said, and it rings true within our present dilemma, "Everybody's not going to make it." We are not inherently pessimistic. Neither are we hyperbolic nor primarily motivated by negative denunciations. Yet, we have come to use the most precise methods of analyzing our status and that of the larger society. This is a bad time in America's civilization journey, and it's hard to point to any point of our own journey of the *Maafa* (the "great suffering") where things have gone particularly well for Blacks.

Our collective backs are pressed against the wall. Yet, within this sense of urgency, we must be decisive, precise, and uncompromising in our resolve to overcome our group's huge pitfalls. Previous generations have faced even worse challenges.

Like so many generations before us, what we do now and for the foreseeable future will largely determine the fate of our people. The stakes are incredibly high. This is a time when we call upon our great saints – the names of Harriet Tubman, Nat Turner, Marcus Garvey, Ida Wells-Barnett, Malcolm X, Martin L. King, Jr., Queen Mother Moore, and many others are sweet on our tongues because of the courageous ways that they confronted adversity.

It's not like we don't have choices. Our Great Ancestors illuminated distinct pathways through the cultural darkness to places where we could find refuge and resilience. The libraries are full of magnificent narratives. We have Wise and Esteemed Elders in our midst to serve as guides. But, in the end, we are truly the masters of our fate – We are the captains of our cultural soul.

The New D.R.O.P. Squad

There's only one fight left—just one – and that's the Fight for the Black mind, and we're losing... We are Losing!

The Greatest pathology in the world, the greatest sickness in the world, is for a people to believe in something just because they wish for it to be so. And that's where most of us are! – Dr. Bobby E. Wright

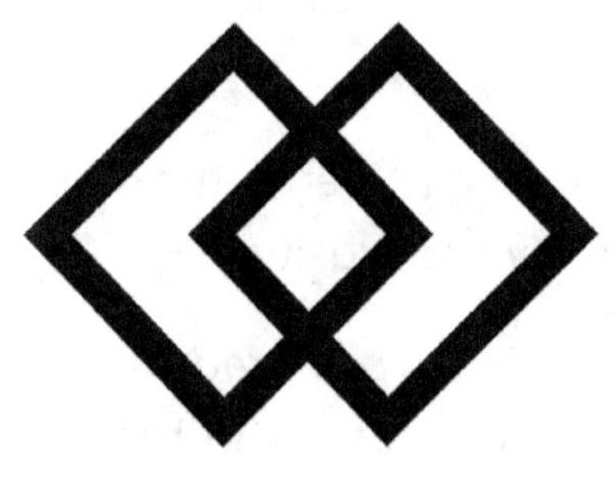

Epa represents handcuffs, a symbol of bondage. The symbol reminds offenders of the uncompromising nature of the law.

In 1994 there was a radical, black-themed movie that captivated the culturally conscious community's attention and excited many conversations about dealing with the excessive amount of compromise, selling out, and "coonish" behavior we were observing in middle-class aspiring black men. That film was ***Drop Squad***, directed by David C. Johnson and starring Eriq La Salle, Vondie Curtis-Hall, and Ving Rhames. The buzz among our more militant brothers was pretty supportive.

A brief synopsis of the film:

Political satire about an underground militant group that kidnaps African-Americans who have sold out their race. The story follows as the group led Curtis-Hall and Rhames kidnaps an advertising executive (La Salle) who has been providing advertising programs that belittle blacks and women. One advertisement features Spike Lee endorsing Gospelpak Fried Chicken which comes in a bucket with the Confederate flag draped all over it.[44]

Some of the relevant highlights of the film included:

- The acronym D.R.O.P. stands for *Deprogramming and Reorientation Of Priorities*:

- The underground Brothers targeted Blacks whom they determined were sellouts to the white-dominated culture at the expense of members of their own ethnic group;

- The movie highlighted commercialized ethnic stereotypes, such as offensive advertisements for fried chicken and malt liquor;

- Also targeted for sarcastic criticism were the hyper-sexualization of women and excessive religiosity;

- Targeted for reprogramming are such *compradors* as ad agency marketers, corrupt politicians, those who turn their backs on opportunities for other Blacks, and sleazy evangelists;

- While the preferred techniques for reprogramming center around mind control programming, some members of the Drop Squad would like to use harsher methods leaning toward torture.

There are many parallels to these themes from the 1990s movie to what we witness today. Perhaps there is a need to revive a strategic demand to deprogram and reprioritize some of the black men of our present generation.

---

[44] Drop Squad Plot, written by John Sacksteder, IMDB

Media Literacy

We have established how ideas are diffused by multiple means of communication and can ultimately become an extension of the culture that guides and impacts the lives of the masses. For decades, I, along with countless associates and comrades, have examined these persuasive conversations and how they have frequently undermined our best interests as a functioning group-within-a-group, Blacks within the Diaspora countries. We have highlighted the impact of empowering and disempowering media and messages across the spectrum of communication platforms ranging from music and theater to radio, television, cinema, commercials, social media, video games, and now virtual reality.

We must have a trained cadre that can decode these messages in real-time, especially those that pose an undermining threat to the integrity of our people's existence, thriving, sovereignty, and sustainable development. Along the way, we have come across many sources revealing insight into how these messages are crafted to have maximum impact on the unwitting targets of persuasion campaigns.

There can be no questioning that our group has been negatively impacted by the significant decline in literacy that has occurred to our members, from the earliest school years even through to senior citizens; Blacks are falling behind other ethnic groups in functional literacy and educational attainment. We are being dumbed down in real-time from generation to generation. This era of pervasive social media triviality isn't compatible with our desire for increased literacy in the population.

The Hidden Persuaders

The 1957 book by Vance Packard, **THE HIDDEN PERSUADERS**, is a masterpiece expose of the many ways that commercial advertisement advanced multiple mechanisms of mind control, persuasion, and the creation of emotional needs during the 20th Century. This is another book I will highly recommend to each of us who is determined to educate ourselves to the highest level of resistance to externally imposed thought manipulation. In a chapter entitled "So Ad Men Become Depth Men, Vance Packard wrote the following regarding the evolution of the sciences of persuasion as advanced by business advertisers:

> The triggers would be needed once the real motivations were diagnosed. They could get guidance on the matter of triggers from Clyde Miller's book *The Process of Persuasion*, where it was pointed out that astute persuaders always use word triggers and picture triggers to evoke desired responses. Once a response pattern is established in terms of persuasion, then you can persuade people in wholesale lots, because all of us, as Professor Miller pointed out, are "creatures of conditioned reflex." In his view, the crux of all persuasion jobs, whether selling soft drinks or a political philosophy, is to develop these conditional reflexes by flashing on trigger words, symbols, or acts.[45]

Looking through my copy of Packard's book, which is extensively highlighted, I find many relevant insights that would seem to have increased in their relevance to the major problems that impact society 65 years after the book's publication. For

---

[45] THE HIDDEN PERSUADERS, by Vance Packard, 1957, pg. 18

example, in the chapter *"Marketing Eight Hidden Needs,"* the author writes:

> The probers found significance in the fact that the home freezer first came into widespread popularity after World War II when many families were filled with inner anxieties because of uncertainties involving not only food but just about everything else in their lives. These people began thinking fondly of former periods of safety and security, which subconsciously took them back to childhood where there was the mother who never disappointed and love was closely related with the giving of food. The probers concluded: "The freezer represents to many the assurance that there is always food in the house, and food in the home represents security, warmth, and safety." People who feel insecure, they found, need more food around than they can eat. The agency decided that the merchandising of freezers should take this squirrel factor into account in shaping campaigns. [Packard 1957, pg. 62]

A Century of Selfishness and Control

We are on a broad mission of deprogramming all self-effacing ideologies from our people that constrain sovereign development and creating a new sense of confidence, competence, and motivation to accomplish. Some impressive efforts in recent years can be seen as powerful, useful tools for reorientating priorities.

One great example of this was a British TV documentary series that can still be seen across the Internet, ***The Century of the Self***:

> The Century of the Self is a 2002 British television documentary series by filmmaker Adam Curtis. It focuses on the work of psychoanalysts Sigmund Freud and Anna Freud, and PR consultant Edward Bernays. In episode one, Curtis says, "This series is about how those in power have used Freud's theories to try and control the dangerous crowd in an age of mass democracy." [Wiki]

This explosive series aired at the beginning of the new century and, as its title implies, forecasts what might be in store for the next 100 years based on multiple trends of mass mind control, social engineering, and the disproportionate usurpation of power by a global elite.

One critic, Zsolt Babocsai, whose synopses of each episode are shared herein, said of the series broadcast in the UK:

> This documentary is nothing short of astonishing. It gives you an explanation to why the world is the way it is today and how human nature shaped it in the past century. Even if you didn't learn any new facts from it (you will), it would be worth watching just for the way it connects the dots. It's made up of four parts.

The series aired in four episodes from March 17-April 7, 2002:

1. **Happiness Machines** – "The film starts with the ideas of Sigmund Freud, who believed that humans are irrational and are governed by their subconscious fears and desires. His nephew, Edward Bernays, put his theory to practice and got to work to build a social structure that controls the masses that could not be trusted to control themselves and would pose a threat otherwise."

2. **The Engineering of Consent** – "Psychoanalysts like [Ernest] Dichter trained corporations to identify and exploit people's fears and desires. By the early 50s their ideas became widely accepted in business as well as politics. The reason why they did what they did was they believed that by regulating people's wild desires and unconscious fears, we'd live in a better society. By giving people products that complement their personalities, products they could identify with, people would become more stable emotionally and able to lead more balanced and happy lives. Psychoanalysts believed that ordinary individuals and the masses were not capable of being democratic by themselves unless their unstable way of being was controlled."

3. **There is a Policeman Inside All Our Heads; He Must Be Destroyed** – "The Freudian view of the human psyche is based on dangerous and primitive emotions and their repression. That's why Anna Freud tried to cure her patients by putting them in a new environment and that's why she died a virgin. Wilhelm Reich believed the opposite. He thought that sexual energy had to be expressed freely to be healthy and that humans are inherently good, but the society that wanted to repress their inner energies made them sick and dangerous. He also believed a lot of baloney, like he could cure cancer and make rain fall... Abraham Maslow and his pyramid of needs provided a basis for business to segment society into groups that had their own desires."

4. **Eight People Sipping Wine in Kettering** – "The first three episodes showed how business learned to read consumers' desires and sell them products that satisfied them. The closing episode shows how politics has done the same towards the end of the century using the very same

techniques as business. In the classic model of politics, different candidates showed up with their different agendas and it was up to the voter to choose one that matched their preferences. In this new system dominated by super granular opinion polls and analysis of people's political desires, each candidate tried to match their agenda to what they thought people wanted."

Twenty years after the series production, it is still highly recommended that every independent thinking person give it a watch. I have viewed each episode several times. I particularly appreciate watching it in the presence of a culturally conscious community. It unquestionably stands as one of our generation's outstanding productions of liberation media.

Mind Control

Aldous Huxley, the author of the 1932 dystopian novel **BRAVE NEW WORLD**, wrote a lesser-known follow-up, published in 1958, **BRAVE NEW WORLD REVISITED**. In the latter book, he looked at many of the futurist projections from his book of 26 years earlier, realizing that he had been profoundly accurate with many of the troubling ideas he wrote about in his younger years. My book **MIND CONTROL: Resistance is Possible** had a chapter entitled *FROM BRAVE NEW WORLD TO NEW WORLD ORDER: Mind Control and the Relevance of the Writings of Aldous Huxley*, within which I examined multiple themes from the noted author, some of which are relevant here.

Huxley wrote about the power of symbols to penetrate our subconscious minds at the individual and societal levels to implant transforming ideas and values:

> Find some common desire, some widespread unconscious fear or anxiety; think out some way to relate this wish or fear to the product you have to sell; then build a bridge of verbal or pictorial symbols over which your customer can pass from fact to compensatory dream, and from the dream to the illusion that your product, when purchased, will make the dream come true.[46]

Huxley further states how increasing psychological stress levels make one more vulnerable to subjection to mind-controlling influences. Considering the saturation of stressing communications, entertainment, and community conditions, along with the tension caused by economic and political problems, we might conclude that Blacks in the U.S. and other diaspora settings are more stressed than others.

> The effectiveness of political and religious propaganda depends upon the methods employed, not upon the doctrines taught. These doctrines may be true or false, wholesome or pernicious – it makes little or no difference. If the indoctrination is given in the right way at the proper state of nervous exhaustion, it will work. Under favorable conditions, practically everybody can be converted to practically anything. [Huxley 1958, pg. 78]

There is much more to comprehend about how mind controllers have established their empires of influence. I highly recommend that all of my **Big Up Manhood** comrades get my book **MIND CONTROL**, and step up your awareness of these techniques deployed against us. <u>Resistance is Possible!</u>

---

[46] BRAVE NEW WORLD REVISITED, by Aldous Huxley, 1958, pg. 63

Mass Media Amplifies Our Ideas in the World

In this chapter, I have strived to expand an understanding of the many ways that cultural media projected through communications initiatives is intended to shape lives and determine widespread patterns of behavior. Media matters. The long-held adage, conveyed in a timeless children's rhyme, has been negated, "Sticks and stones may break my bones, but words will never hurt me" – that is very far from true.

I've highlighted the ultimate impact of manipulative words projected across the global society, especially by those would-be controllers whose self-interests clash with our natural birthrights. We have a solemn and sacred duty to seek freedom, dignity, self-determination, and sovereign and sustainable development for our future generations. Instead, these manipulators have made their ideologies intergenerational, teaching their sons and daughters to control entire segments of a vulnerable population for all time.

The same mechanisms that enable these manipulators of the truth to project their vile doctrines upon society are accessible to those of us who are aligned with liberation and the highest expression of humanity. We outnumber the controllers, yet they have seized upon many means of amplifying their ideas through the deft use of mass communications of all forms:

- Print media in the form of books, magazines, flyers, newspapers, journals, newsletters, posters, comic books, and billboards;

- Broadcast media such as terrestrial radio, television, Internet webcasting, cable television, and drama programming;

- Live entertainment performances such as concerts, theater, musicals, nightclubs, drum and dance groups;

- Cinema, documentaries, animation, view-on-demand streaming media, and DVDs;

- Town hall meetings, community gatherings, speaker platforms, panel discussions, and public engagements of all sorts;

- Person-to-person, word-of-mouth information sharing.

We have many of their operational formulas in our possession, such as the following precise formula for social engineering:

"Sufficient financial backing for regular utilization of mass media, constantly to communicate the desired objectives to the 'common man.' New values can be deliberately created, disseminated, and adopted as personal and collective goals highly desirable of achievement. But the concerted effort of the major social institutions—particularly the educational, recreational, and religious—must be enlisted with the ready cooperation of those in control of the mass media... By utilizing the various tested devices, our modern genius in advertising may alight upon simple phrases well organized in sequence and timing, and coordinated with other efforts geared to realize the 'grand design.' But there are required a host of laborers with plenty of financial backing.

"In mapping out his "grand design" for making us all more dutiful consumers he accepted, without any question that I could note, the basic assumption that achieving the one-third-better goal was worth any manipulating that might be necessary to achieve It."[47]

I have had the opportunity to collect many such formulaic strategies to manipulate and control societies and am proud to have been able to expose these in the four dozen books I have written. But, beyond mere collection and comprehension of such, I am committed to expanding this awareness to as many who would accept these insights and get excited about using them to project liberty, equality, and dignity.

We live in a spectacular time in the history of civilizations. We stand at a crossroads separating the previous 2600 years of a history of humiliation, encroachment, cultural colonization, mass genocide, and many crimes against the humanity of African people on this planet – separating that sordid past from a dawning of a new era in global history where we rise like the symbolic Phoenix from the ashes. Africa Rising is the flaming banner we thrust into the skies above our people. This transformation is the most significant paradigm shift affecting our people in the past 600 years.

It is truly an honor and a privilege to have this **Big Up Manhood** confront these challenges and those we will continue to face.

We are truly Great People. As Marcus Garvey admonished, we "have a glorious history." We stand at the doorstep of the next greatest chapter in our people's long record of accomplishments.

It is fitting that we conclude with the words of our Great Ancestor, Marcus Garvey, speaking in Harlem circa 1924:

---

[47] Sociologist Philip J. Allen, Univ. of Virginia, cited in THE HIDDEN PERSUADERS, by Vance Packard, 1957, pg. 261

Well, I intend, with your help and God's grace, to continue; cause my work has only just begun. And future generations shall have in their hands the guide by which they shall know the sins of the 20th century. I know, and I know you to believe in time, but we shall wait patiently for 200 years if need be, to face our enemies through our posterity. When mine enemies are satisfied, in life, I shall come back or in death even to serve you as I served before. In life, I shall be the same; in death, I SHALL BE A TERROR to foes of African liberty.

If death hath power, then count on me to be the real Marcus Garvey I would like to be. If I may come in an earthquake, or a plague, or a pestilence, or as God would have me, then be assured that I shall never desert you and make your enemies triumph over you. Will I yet not go to hell a million times for you? If I die in Atlanta, my work will only just then begin. For I shall live in the physical or the spiritual to see the day of Africa's Glory.

When I am dead, wrap the mantle of the Red, the Black and the Green around me for in a New Life I shall RISE UP with God's grace and blessings to lead the millions to the heights of triumph that you well know. Look for me in the whirlwind or a storm; look for me all around you, for with God's grace, I shall come back with countless millions of Black men and women who have died in America, those who have died in the West Indies and those who have died in Africa to aid You in the fight for liberty, freedom and life.

... Let NO ONE inoculate you with evil doctrines to suit his own conveniences. "Charity begins at home." So first to thyself be true and "thou canst not then be false to no man."

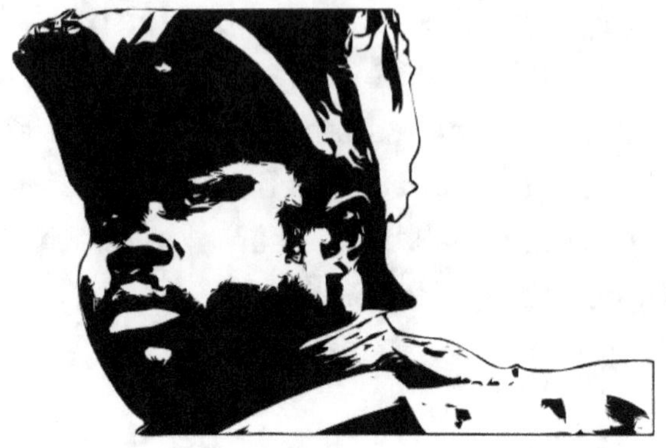

BIBLIOGRAPHY

Books to Read on These Topics

THE ROAD TO POWER: Seven Steps to an African Global Order – Keidi Obi Awadu (1999)

LIVING SUPERFOOD LONGEVITY: Mastering the Possibilities of High Quality Life Extension – Keidi Obi Awadu (2016)

FURIOUSLY VEGAN: 221 Steps to Restore Youthful Vitality – Keidi Obi Awadu (2021)

MISSING ASSETS: Cultural, Biological, and Psychological Origins of Infertility – Keidi Obi Awadu (1997

LIVING SUPERFOOD LONGEVITY: Master the Possibilities of High-Quality Life Extension – Keidi Obi Awadu (2016

HE NEW SCRAMBLE FOR AFRICA – Keidi Obi Awadu (2015)

MAN HEAL THYSELF: The Wellness Warrior's Journey to Self-Mastery – Supanova Slom and Queen Afua (2021)

THE CLASH OF CIVILIZATION: And the Remaking of World Order – Samuel P. Huntington, 1996

POPULATION DECLINE AND THE REMAKING OF GREAT POWER POLITICS – Susan Yoshihara and Douglas A. Sylva (2012)

INTERNATIONAL ASPECTS OF OVER-POPULATION: Proceedings of a Conference held by the South African Institute of International Affairs – Edited by John Baratt and Michael Luow (1972)

AN AMERICAN DILEMMA: The Negro Problem and Modern Democracy – Gunnar Myrdal (1944)

SILENT SPRING – Rachael Carson (1962)

OUR STOLEN FUTURE: Are We Threatening our Fertility, Intelligence, and Survival? – Theo Colborn, Dianne Dumanoski, and John Peterson Myers (1996)

THE GREAT PROSTATE HOAX: How Big Medicine Hijacked the PSA Test and Caused a Public Health Disaster – Dr. Richard J. Ablin with Ronald Piana (2014)

BLUEPRINT FOR BLACK POWER: A Moral, Political, and Economic Imperative for the Twenty-First Century – Amos Wilson (1998)

Further Resources

Hormones are key in brain health differences between men and women, by Laura Williamson, American Heart Association News, Feb 1, 2021 -
https://www.heart.org/en/news/2021/02/01/hormones-are-key-in-brain-health-differences-between-men-and-women

Female Hormone Key to Male Brain, by David Biello, Scientific American, January 4, 2006 -
https://www.scientificamerican.com/article/female-hormone-key-to-mal/

Sex in the Brain: Genes, Hormones, and Evolution, by Anita Devineni, Brains Explained, March 14, 2015 -
https://www.brains-explained.com/sex-in-the-brain/

INDEX